Praise for
Joyful, Delicious, Vegan:
Life Without Heart Disease

"*Joyful, Delicious, Vegan: Life Without Heart Disease* is an inspiring guide to achieving the very best of health. The power of foods is surprising— even life-changing—and this immensely practical book will guide you to putting it to use."

—NEAL D. BARNARD, MD, FACC, Adjunct Professor, George Washington University School of Medicine, and president of Physicians Committee for Responsible Medicine

"The late Malcom X once stated that 'Black women in the United States have historically been under the greatest attack in our society.' After practicing cardiology for more than twenty years, I have come to know firsthand that the greatest threat to our Black women has been heart disease. We are literally at war. However, we are also blessed with brave warriors like Sherra Aguirre. In *Joyful, Delicious, Vegan: Life Without Heart Disease*, Sherra outlines a powerful, effective battle plan to defeat heart disease. This must-read book serves as both an inspiring health journey and a stepwise health guide for anyone battling heart disease or any other chronic illness."

—BAXTER MONTGOMERY, MD, FACC, Clinical Assistant Professor of Medicine, Division of Cardiology/Cardiac Electrophysiology, University of Texas Health Science Center, Houston and Medical Director Montgomery Heart and Wellness

"Sherra Aguirre has written a thoughtful, well-researched book that combines nutrition science, medicine and her personal inner awareness, and which will serve our community well in this era of rapid transformation. May her words resonate with you in your journey toward optimum health and global well-being."

—SAILESH RAO, PhD, systems specialist, founder of Climate Healers, author of *Carbon Yoga: The Vegan Metamorphosis* and executive producer of *Cowspiracy, The Sustainability Secret,* and *What the Health*

"A great health resource for everyone concerned with our deteriorating health in a world of scientific advances that should be improving it, this book is a journey back to health by going back to basics—by recognizing, appreciating, and returning the love of our body's highly evolved 60 trillion cells, which work hard 24/7 to keep us healthy. It shows us our own ability to heal disease by paying absolute attention to what we are feeding them, by changing our diets in ways that ensure their well-being."

—ELISABET SAHTOURIS, PhD, evolution biologist, futurist, and author of *Gaia's Dance: The Story of Earth and Us*

j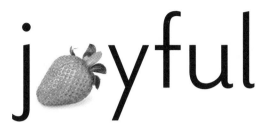yful

delicious
vegan

life without
heart disease

Sherra Aguirre

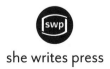

she writes press

Published 2021
Printed in the United States of America
Print ISBN: 978-1-64742-063-5
E-ISBN: 978-1-64742-064-2
Library of Congress Control Number: 2020917546

For information, address:
She Writes Press
1569 Solano Ave #546
Berkeley, CA 94707

Interior design by Tabitha Lahr
Interior illustrations © Shutterstock.com

She Writes Press is a division of SparkPoint Studio, LLC.

All company and/or product names may be trade names, logos, trademarks, and/or registered trademarks and are the property of their respective owners.

Names and identifying characteristics have been changed to protect the privacy of certain individuals.

This book is dedicated to my mother, Odell Christine Sweats Johnson, my first love, whose quiet grace as she battled Alzheimer's disease taught me how precious are the gifts of life and health.

Medical Disclaimer

THE INFORMATION IN THIS BOOK is intended to be of help in regaining or maintaining good health overall and heart health in particular, and to help readers improve their diet, lifestyle, and approach to self-care. It is not intended to diagnose, treat, or otherwise replace medical advice from a physician or other health care provider. You should always consult your physician for the diagnosis or treatment of any condition, and before making any changes to current treatments or medications, including recommendations contained in this book. The author and publisher are not liable for the treatment or outcomes from any specific conditions or illnesses. Please do not delay seeking medical attention because of anything you read in this book or in any of its reference materials. The references and source materials in this book are intended to provide additional helpful information and do not constitute an endorsement of those works or websites. Please also be advised that websites referenced are subject to change.

Contents

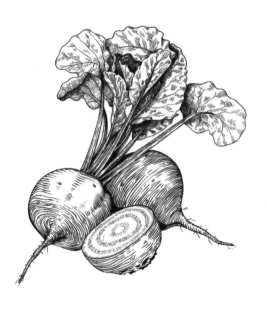

Introduction

WHAT IF YOU HAD THE POWER to remain disease free by feeding your health instead of your illness? How would you feel if the person in charge of your care fed you unhealthy food and, when you got sick, fed you drugs along with more unhealthy food? Or when your health continued to deteriorate, what if they gave you more drugs and the same unhealthy food? This is exactly what we do to ourselves. I believe that without a nutritious, plant-strong diet, we undermine our body's harmony with our natural environment, its balance, and its ability to keep us well. *Everything we need to stay healthy is available to us, and it starts in our own kitchens.* Doctors, health care practitioners, and others can assist us, but in this book, I will show you how your own everyday choices can have the biggest impact on your wellness and quality of life.

By choosing to feed our health and not our illness, we demonstrate gratitude and love for this wondrous human body we are fortunate enough to inhabit for a time. We set in motion a chain of positive events—physical, biological, emotional, and spiritual—that are life enhancing and life changing. Becoming more mindful of this power to transform our lives and heal our bodies is a turning point in reclaiming our health and joy of living. By doing so, we can heal our broken connection to our natural environment and reclaim the good health that this connection provides.

HEALTH CRISES FUELED BY THE STANDARD AMERICAN DIET (SAD)

Have you ever wondered why almost everyone you know is suffering—or has friends or family members suffering—from diabetes, high blood pressure, heart disease, or cancer? Have you noticed the increase in advertising in the media for "maintenance" drugs and other pharmaceuticals compared to five or ten years ago? When did dialysis clinics begin to pop up in our communities like McDonald's franchises?

We are witnessing a health care crisis of epidemic proportions whose reach and devastation for individuals, families, and communities is increasing at an alarming rate. The leading cause of death for African Americans, Hispanics, whites, and most other groups in the US is heart disease according to the CDC. In America, nearly half of all adults are living with some form of cardiovascular disease, which includes forty-six percent of African American men.[1] Forty-nine percent of African American women are affected, and black women are nearly twice as likely to have a stroke as white women.[2] Twenty percent are more likely to die from all causes of the disease.[3]

The outlook for diabetes is no better. In a February 2020 National Diabetes Statistics Report update, the CDC reported that over thirty-two million adults have diabetes, with an additional eighty-eight million adults who are prediabetic, for a total of 45 percent of the US population.[4] African Americans are currently twice as likely as non-Hispanic whites to be diagnosed, and African American women were twice as likely to die from diabetes in 2017.[5] Nearly forty million people in the US are projected to be diagnosed as diabetic by 2030.[6] This is a serious problem for families and for the health care system, despite the fact that Type 2 diabetes is both preventable and curable through diet and lifestyle changes.

We cannot watch TV or browse the internet without seeing ad after ad promoting "maintenance" medicines to manage the symptoms of heart disease, diabetes, and other chronic diseases without curing any of them. The same big food and drug companies that offer a food supply engineered with added fat, sugar, salt, chemicals, and additives to drive sales and high profits, also supply and profit from the maintenance drugs we must rely on to live with the resulting damage to our bodies.

Diseases like diabetes, high blood pressure, and cancer are fueled by what I like to call the "industrial age diet." It is a diet rooted in conditions from another time and place. It is surrounded by both nostalgia and tradition, which make it difficult to see that, although many foods may look and even taste like the foods we grew up with, they can be very different in origin and nutritional content. They are often genetically altered, have traces of toxic pesticides, and contain artificial flavor enhancers, preservatives, or other chemical additives almost always found in processed foods.

FOOD AS CURE

I began my own food and wellness journey about forty years ago when I started to struggle to stay alert and to focus in the afternoon after eating my usual fast food lunch. I didn't give much thought to the typical American staples of my diet, which included lots of fried chicken, barbecue, burgers, and fries. I started to notice that about an hour after a quick lunch at whichever fast food place was most convenient, my energy would drop through the floor, and I would drag myself through the rest of the afternoon. I was young enough not to have experienced other negative health effects from my lifestyle and food choices. I simply noticed the connection between what I ate for lunch and how I felt afterwards and decided to take action.

I didn't make a radical change. I just cut back little by little on fried, heavy, highly processed foods. And I felt better, so much so that it sparked an interest in the effects of diet on health, as well as a lifelong commitment to myself. Each year, I made small changes which had positive and cumulative effects on my health and wellness, and over time these changes would reshape my outlook on life.

For the next two decades, as I learned more about health and food, I adopted a primarily vegetarian diet. And then in my fifties, I began to experience the cardiovascular issues and hypertension with which my family struggled. I knew I had to do more and adopted a wholly plant-based/vegan diet. My body guided me along the journey through the ups and downs of prescription drugs and their negative side effects, to eating healing foods and experiencing positive side effects. When my body spoke, I learned to listen and discovered that there was usually a natural solution for most of my challenges.

Over time, I began to experience my body differently. A profound love and respect grew within me for each part, each cell, and for what I like to call our internal ecosystem, by whose innate "intelligence" we are offered the opportunity for good health. This gratitude for the health with which I have been blessed, and for the growing body of knowledge about the amazing intelligence coded into our cells, our food and Earth itself, has been both humbling and empowering.

JOURNEY TOWARD GRATITUDE AND ABUNDANCE

This book is about the adventure, fun, and spiritual fulfillment of eating and living consciously. It shows us how thinking differently and taking action on how we feed ourselves leads to empowerment and connection with the natural abundance that food represents. The realization that there are solutions to our most common health problems and that the very same solutions meaningfully impact our environmental problems—that we are not powerless in the face of either—is life changing. Even the smallest steps we take toward a

> How we choose, interact with, prepare, and eat our food can improve our health, communities, and the health of our planet. It can and will save lives, and it starts in our own kitchens.

having bigger view of ourselves and our relationship to the natural world in which we live will help tip the scales (pun intended) in our favor.

I have always thought of the saying "you are what you eat" in physical terms. I now realize the meaning goes much deeper. How and what we eat not only determines our health, but our mood, attitude, energy, and how we experience the world. Mindful eating is transformational. It will shape the legacy we leave our children. These are the things that compelled me to write this book. In doing so I join the growing chorus of voices from all walks of life who have decided to take charge of their health. Our lives and the lives of those we love depend on it.

I am very grateful for the holistic health care practitioners, physicians, and all of those who have advocated and shared natural health and traditional healing wisdom. I am also grateful for those who have added to those ancient healing traditions the knowledge from scientific study we now have available to us. Most of all, I am grateful for every single cell in my body that loves me unconditionally and guides me toward better health with its functional intelligence. *I want you to know how you too can experience this feeling of love and gratitude to propel you on your own food journey to great health, vibrancy, and connection.*

Along with my own, I will share success stories about other people who have experienced a reversal of diabetes, heart disease, and other diet- and lifestyle-related illnesses. I want you to have useful information from scientific studies and hear from cutting-edge lifestyle medical experts that point to diet as the underlying cause of these diseases and the dietary changes that can reverse them. And most importantly, I want each of you to have the resources, tools, tips, and recipes to create a healthier and more joyful life for yourself and those you love.

We will look at how combining healing whole foods with other lifestyle changes—like mindfulness, surrounding ourselves with people who support us, engaging in more physical activity, and choosing how we respond to stress—can provide results that are nothing short of amazing. The changes we make radiate outward to make our communities, all life, and Earth itself healthier. They also help us to live with more love and compassion as we experience gratitude for delicious and life-giving whole plant foods, and a greater connection to the simple beauty and abundance of life all around us. When this love is acknowledged it compels us to reciprocate, and its healing effects are powerful!

Let's get started.

part 1:
the foundation

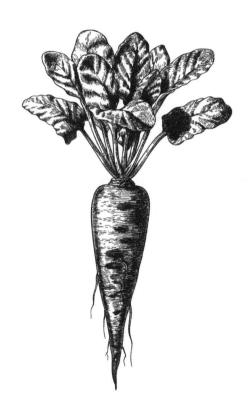

CHAPTER 1:

Listen and Love—Living and Feeding Ourselves Mindfully

"The greatest medicine of all is teaching people how not to need it."
—HIPPOCRATES, father of modern medicine, fifth century BC

"SHOW YOUR HEARTBURN WHO'S BOSS!" says the actress in an acid reflux commercial, which suggests that by taking this particular antacid product, you can continue to "enjoy" the same foods that contributed to the problem in the first place. In our media-dominated, consumer-based society, we are coaxed into viewing our body as the simple servant of the brain. The messages and images we hear and see all around us tell us how this servant should behave and what it should look and feel like. We are happy if ours fits the popular definition of beautiful or strong, and if it carries us through our daily activities without demanding too much of our attention. However, when contrary to our expectations, it is too fat or too thin or begins to experience pain or discomfort, we want to fix the problem quickly so the body can do its job without complaint, and we can get on with whatever it is we think is more important.

Western medicine, which was born in the industrial age, frames this view by treating the body as a machine that is the sum of its parts, not a highly complex, interdependent, and intelligent energy system. In this view, communication is one way—top down. Only recently have mainstream health care providers begun to consider the mind/body/spirit connection in their treatment methods. We have all heard stories about people, quite often the elderly, who are prescribed one medication for this, another for that, and yet another for the side effects of the first two. A friend of mine was asked to take an elderly neighbor whose health was in decline to her doctor's visit. He rounded up her eleven prescribed medications to take to the appointment. Not only was her primary care provider unaware of some of the medications, which had been prescribed by specialists, he discovered many of her health problems were actually side effects from drug interactions. It has been stated by geriatric specialists that many symptoms commonly experienced by the elderly actually stem from drug interactions compounded by poor diet and often depression. And of course, the pharmaceutical industry has prescriptions for that too!

UNCONDITIONAL LOVE

I want to paint for you a very different picture of the complex and intelligent energy field we simply think of as our body. About eleven years ago, I decided to spend a week at a health and detox spa in the California desert. I was fighting burnout at work and coping with the recent death of my mother. Little did I know that I would meet someone who would forever change the way I thought about my health. Susana Belen, the founder of We Care Spa, was the most energetic sixty-something-year-old I had ever met. Her petite frame, personal warmth, and flaming red hair made her a standout among the staff whenever she taught yoga and nutrition classes.

During one of her sessions, she shared a powerful metaphor. Susana asked us to visualize the trillions of cells in our bodies, each of which faithfully performs a very specific function necessary for our health. Each of these tiny, microscopic entities exists for no other reason than to promote our well-being according to its functional "intelligence." She spoke with a quiet passion about their unconditional love for and devotion to us in a way that made me believe I could feel that love.

That night in my small cabin, after my evening meditation, I started to sob and could not stop. The stresses of my work and the loss of my mother had weighed heavily on me for months, and I realized that coming to this place and meeting Susana was part of my healing process.

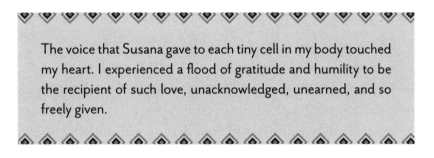

The voice that Susana gave to each tiny cell in my body touched my heart. I experienced a flood of gratitude and humility to be the recipient of such love, unacknowledged, unearned, and so freely given.

Because I am now aware of this wondrous intelligence within me and in every one of us—in every living creature, and Earth itself—I want to return this love each and every day.

I now feel a sense of responsibility and teamwork with the cells that make up my physical body. I know that if I eat poorly, expose my body to toxins (environmental or ingested), deprive it of rest, and subject it to high stress levels, my cells struggle to protect me. At some point they try to get my attention—a mild headache, upset stomach, or low energy, perhaps so slight that I hardly notice. Before I became aware that this was their way to communicate with me, whenever these mild distress signals appeared, my first thought was simply to stop the discomfort. Like that commercial actress, I would take a painkiller or whatever over-the-counter remedy was available. Usually the symptoms would go away, and I'd return to my normal activities again without giving the matter much thought. By not taking the time to listen more closely to my body's messages, I missed many opportunities to understand how my choices and actions were undercutting my health. I also missed opportunities to make early changes to practice better self-care. My cells worked harder to keep me well, and with the symptoms gone, it was easy for me to continue making the same food and lifestyle choices that compromised them in the first place. The behavior of our cells is the very definition of unconditional love!

LEARNING TO LISTEN

It is the norm in our culture to live life in this way. With our symptoms abated or managed, we go on with life as usual until the body's distress signals can no longer be ignored or silenced with over-the-counter drugs. At some point, taking action can no longer be deferred, and we get the bad news that we will now have to deal with a life-changing condition or event. And, depending on the nature or severity of the diagnosis, our tiny cells that have labored tirelessly to keep us from arriving at this point, that tried to tell us what they needed, will now be subjected to a medical intervention that will help some of them and perhaps disrupt or harm others. And then we face the risk of a downward health spiral that might have been avoided by paying attention, by listening and making changes when the messages were gentle, and the problem was small.

I now know how important it is to recognize and to be mindful of the aches, pains, and twinges that are messages from this cellular love so unconditionally given. The body is programmed to keep us well if we feed it a healthy diet, pay attention to how it reacts to the choices we make, and follow its lead. My goal now is to set a very different chain of events in motion. If I have heartburn, I first look at what may be contributing to the problem. Then I allow myself to feel empathy and love for the cells that make up my esophagus and digestive tract. I put the discomfort I feel in the context of the greater distress they must feel. I imagine how difficult it must be for them to utilize some of the foods I eat that lack nutrients they need to protect my health. I also remind myself that the only thing that can heal any illness is my body itself. Drugs, surgery, and other treatments can assist, but the body does the healing, not the drugs or the doctors! And I acknowledge that each food and lifestyle choice I make either feeds my health or feeds an illness, regardless of any medications I may take to control my symptoms.

Every action we take, however small, has both direct and indirect effects. Every choice we make either brings us more in harmony with our desires and intentions or moves us toward some other result or outcome. It either reinforces old habits or establishes new ones. We don't have to be perfect, and the good news is that we get many opportunities to realign our actions with our best intentions. Life offers us many "do overs," and for this we can all be very thankful. Because the body is so resilient, we can make small positive steps over time to feed our wellness and open a pathway to a result very different from the downward spiral described earlier. However, at some point the do overs end, and we see the result of an accumulation of our choices, both conscious and unconscious.

THE POWER

The German term *gestalt* refers to the principle that the whole is greater than the sum of its parts. It is a simple but very appropriate term to describe our body and how it works, and why making an attentive, loving, and thoughtful choice in response to something as simple as heartburn will reverberate throughout our system in subtle ways we may not immediately feel.

We are not machines but living, breathing, loving masses of intelligent energy, connected to the energy and intelligence of nature. Now that I am mindful of the work that my cells do to keep me healthy and see that work as an expression of love, I feel empathy and acknowledge the distress I can cause them with poor everyday choices. My motivations to make better choices are gratitude, love, and the power of knowing what my body is capable of achieving.

Loving choices are powerful. When we are tuned in to our bodies, an ache, pain, or other "problem" is really an alert that offers a pathway to improvements in how well our bodies function. The cells of every organ are connected by energy exchanges with the cells of other parts of the body, and when there is distress or improvement in any one part, it is communicated to and affects the whole. Because of this, our smallest healthy choices have a powerful multiplier effect and can boost our vitality and resilience in surprising ways.

Rather than showing our body "who's the boss," we can direct our efforts to finding the root cause or causes of our symptoms. In the case of acid reflux, we could research it online or consult a health care professional about likely causes or triggers, and to help us rule out the possibility that it may be linked to a more serious condition. We may also speak with a nutritionist about foods that contribute to heartburn, learn about herbal support for healthy digestion, or simply make time to relax with a cup of chamomile tea. *By following this path, we increase the chance that long before more serious distress signals or symptoms appear, we will be on a path to restoration and a natural state of internal harmony, balance, and coherence.*

The concept of coherence is very important and refers to the alignment of our intentions and the food we put into our mouths.

Foods are forms of energy, as are our physical selves. When we pay attention to the signals we get while or after eating our food—lower or higher energy, upset stomach, heartburn, better or poorer ability to focus—that information can help us align what we feed ourselves with our physical needs. By doing so, we help our body to carry out an intention for healthy digestion, for example, with foods that have the nutrients and other attributes (e.g. less fat and sugar) to achieve that result. The food and our body will be able to communicate effectively and work in harmony. Coherence also refers to the emotional or psychological aspect of eating. When we are guided by the body's messages and feed ourselves in concert with that information, we produce a symphony as opposed to energetic discord and noise. The positive results we see and feel will lift our mood and our energy, and will reinforce those actions, which is how new healthy habits are formed. The opportunity for this sequence of events is exactly what our cells, through the symptoms we experience, are communicating to us. If only we would listen and act out of love in return! Unlike the alternative offered by our antacid commercial actress, this is real love.

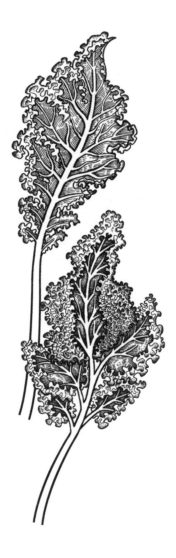

CHAPTER 2:

Eat Your Way to
a Healthy Heart

"Connection is health. And what our society does its best to disguise from us is how ordinary, how commonly attainable, health is. We lose our health—and create profitable diseases and dependencies—by failing to see the direct connections between living and eating, eating and working, working and loving."

—WENDELL BERRY, author and farmer, 2002

STUDIES AND PROVEN RESULTS

In many parts of the world that we call "developing countries," the basic diets of the people who live there have not changed significantly in the last hundred years or more. Heart disease, diabetes, obesity, and common cancers are rare or nonexistent. Some forty or fifty years ago, this intrigued health researchers, public health professionals, and cardiologists who wanted to understand why these diseases were on the rise in the US, and more importantly, the root causes of these diseases and how to prevent them.

Research led to a growing consensus that areas of the world where the populations were essentially free of heart disease had at least one characteristic in common: a mostly plant-based diet with very limited amounts of meat and processed foods. Researchers discovered that as countries began to develop and gain access to industrially processed foods with added fat, salt, sugar, and other chemical substances typical of our Western diet, these diseases began to appear, even though physical activity levels had not changed.

One of the most prominent research projects, published as *The China Study*, was conducted by Dr. T. Colin Campbell and associates at Cornell University in a twenty-year partnership with Oxford University and the Chinese Academy of Preventative Medicine. It has been described as the most comprehensive study of health and nutrition ever conducted.[7]

◇◇◇◇◇◇◇◇◇◇◇◇◇

The conclusions of the China Study were a significant step forward in understanding how diet either kept people healthy or made them sick. This and other research was utilized by cardiologists like Dr. Caldwell Esselstyn and Dr. Dean Ornish, who were distinguished in their field but frustrated with the shortcomings of the traditional approach of drug therapies and surgeries. They were trained to address symptoms but had nothing to offer patients to prevent or cure heart disease. They began to develop their own treatment plans to give patients the knowledge and support to cure themselves. The patients who participated in their studies or followed their plans not only saw marked improvement or reversal of their cardiovascular symptoms, but experienced similar improvements in their overall health, including reducing or eliminating the need for medications for diabetes and other chronic diseases.[8]

Other significant landmark studies include the Adventist Health Study that began in 2002 and included ninety-six thousand people ages 30–112 from all fifty US states and Canada. The participants included 48 percent non-vegetarians, 44 percent vegetarians and semi-vegetarians (ate dairy, eggs, occasional fish/meat/poultry), and 8 percent vegan or entirely plant based.

The European Prospective Investigation into Cancer and Nutrition at Oxford University, also called the EPIC study, which includes sixty-five thousand participants in the UK, began in 1993 and is ongoing. Its findings are that vegans consumed the most fiber and the least amount of saturated fat and overall fat. Vegans also had the lowest systolic and diastolic blood pressure levels, even as compared to vegetarians who eat eggs and dairy. Compared to meat eaters, they had the healthiest body weights and cholesterol levels.[10]

In addition to these very large long-term studies, short-term studies show how quickly the body begins to respond to what we eat. A very interesting one was presented at the 2016 International Conference on Nutrition in Medicine in Washington, DC. In the study, twenty men from Pittsburgh and twenty men from South Africa "traded diets." The Pittsburgh group ate a typical South African diet of black-eyed peas, maize, okra, tomatoes, spinach, mangoes, and pineapple. The South African group ate pancakes, meatloaf, hamburgers, and fries, which are popular in Pittsburgh. After only two weeks, an analysis showed that their gut bacteria were remarkably different. The South African group eating the average Pittsburgh diet "experienced inflammation in the bowel and a 400 percent increase in the secretion of carcinogenic secondary bile acids." In contrast, the Pittsburgh group eating the healthier

South African diet saw an increase in anti-inflammatory markers and reduced carcinogenic secondary bile acids. The study concluded that high fiber levels in the plant-based diet "increases gut bacteria that reduce inflammation, improve blood sugar control, enhance nutrient absorption, and increase fatty acid metabolism, which reduces total fat storage."[11]

INTRODUCTION TO NUTRITION-BASED CURES

The evidence is overwhelmingly clear that eating a wide variety of mostly whole plant foods is the best way to stay healthy or get healthy. That said, there are a lot of special interest groups that spend a lot of money on disinformation or misinformation about food when it threatens their bottom line.

Big agricultural corporations, the meat and dairy industry, and pharmaceutical companies are certainly not interested in losing their profits. They want us to buy their products, and lots of them. As a result, our health care system is straining under the weight of lifestyle- and diet-related diseases, with no end in sight without major change.

In the words of Dr. Caldwell Esselstyn, "We have to turn off the faucet instead of mopping up the floor."

FAMILY HISTORY IS NOT DESTINY

I want to share my personal struggle with heart disease and hypertension, which is called the "silent killer" because there are often no symptoms to alert us that we may be in danger of a life-threatening stroke or heart attack. Heart disease is a condition that affects millions of people and is common among African Americans. In my early thirties, I began eating a primarily vegetarian diet, maintained a healthy weight, and exercised regularly, which I believed would help me avoid the high blood pressure, stroke, and other health risks with which my family members struggled. I continued to make gradual improvements in my diet and lifestyle over the next two decades, such as eliminating fried foods, reducing the number of processed foods I ate, and adding yoga and meditation.

Despite my lifestyle and diet improvements, by my early fifties, my blood pressure started to creep upward. By then, heart disease had taken a toll on my family. For as far back as I could remember, my parents had been on high blood pressure medications. My maternal grandmother battled hypertension and had a stroke in her early seventies, which resulted in a partial paralysis of her left hand. My grandfather died of a massive heart attack in his mid-fifties.

During a recent visit with my cousin Pam, we recounted her mother's lifelong battle with high blood pressure that led to kidney damage and death from kidney failure. Her father, my paternal uncle, who had hypertension and a pacemaker, experienced five heart attacks, the last of which took his life, while he also fought cancer. We lost an aunt from a simultaneous stroke and heart attack, and now our generation is experiencing the same symptoms and warning signs, including the two of us and many of our cousins. Collectively, our family members have had diagnoses of arteriosclerosis, hypertension, enlarged hearts, heart failure, stroke, and aneurysms starting in our fifties or earlier.

Some of the deaths were sudden and untimely. A younger cousin with hypertension worked as an officer in a correctional facility and was married with two young sons. His high blood pressure was thought to be under control, and he seemed to be healthy otherwise, when he came home from work one day with a bad headache. His wife told us he went to bed early, and a few hours later he was unconscious when she went in to check on him. She called an ambulance, but by the time he reached the hospital, he had died.

His blood pressure had suddenly dropped, perhaps from a ruptured aneurysm, which might also explain the sudden severe headache.

At this point in our visit, Pam and I paused to look at each other, and I knew we were both remembering another story that had shaken our entire family to its core. Shortly after the death of this cousin, Pam's younger brother, Wayne, and his wife, Sally, were on their way to a Colorado ski trip they had looked forward to for some time. They were an active and enthusiastic couple in their mid-forties. Wayne had been on medication for high blood pressure for a few years, and it was also thought to be under control. They were running late when they arrived at the airport for their flight. Because Sally worked for an airline company, she went through the security checkpoint quickly, but Wayne took longer. He told her to go ahead to the gate and that he would be right behind her as soon as he cleared.

After a few minutes at the gate, she thought he must have been detained for some reason. Backtracking through the terminal in the direction of the checkpoint, she saw a small crowd gathering in the middle of the concourse. She described a knot in her stomach when she didn't see her husband anywhere. She began to work her way through and around the crowd to get back to security. When she made her way to the front, to her horror, there lay her husband on the floor. He had been rushing to catch up with her when he collapsed with a heart attack at forty-six—his first. He died on the spot.

This was heartbreaking for all the family, and most especially for Pam. Because of the early deaths of her parents and a younger sister, she and Wayne were the only two surviving members of their immediate family. Now there was one.

Pam had been a smoker for more than twenty years and had already undergone a cardiovascular surgical procedure to open a clogged artery and insert a stent. Even after Wayne's sudden death, it was difficult for her to make and sustain the lifestyle changes that her doctors and family members urged her to make. She often made it clear that only she would decide if, when, or how she stopped smoking. I sometimes wondered if she felt there was no use.

Pam did quit smoking, and for good, over ten years ago. She also changed her food habits to eat more fresh fruits and vegetables and less meat, dairy, and processed foods. She started exercising regularly, first walking and then joining a gym. She lost weight and even began working with a trainer. Her doctor is very happy with her results, as she has eliminated or reduced most of her medications. Now she is a beautiful, vibrant, energetic seventy-two-year-old, who has surpassed the life span of her parents and siblings. Pam is writing a new chapter in the health history of our extended family, one that we will pass on to our children, grandchildren, and beyond. She is a living example of what medical researchers have proven: heredity is not as important as making the choice to do what it takes to be healthy, and our body has a remarkable ability to respond!

MY OWN STRUGGLE

I was in denial for months until my doctor finally insisted I start taking medication to lower my blood pressure, and thereby prevent damage to my heart and arteries and the possibility of a stroke. I actually mourned the day I first filled the prescription. And then, after taking the medication for a week or so, I started to feel light-headed from time to time in the evenings. At one point, I went outside to do some work in the yard, and when I quickly got up to go back inside, I felt I was about to faint. I would later learn by checking my blood pressure morning and night that my readings were consistently ten to twenty points lower in the evening. And because I've never been to a doctor's office for a night appointment, the dosage had been calibrated around my morning readings. At night, my blood pressure would drop so low that I was afraid I would pass out. That experience, combined with an occasional racing heartbeat and an episode during which I felt like I might lose consciousness while driving on the freeway, were all scary enough to spur me to seek a food and exercise solution for my hypertension. I set a goal to make my cardiovascular system healthier, achieve normal blood pressure levels, and eventually eliminate the drugs and their side effects.

Although the side effects from the medication were a frightening incentive, the truth was that deep down I believed I could do better. It took longer than I anticipated, and there were ups and downs, including a period in which I thought I would give up because I couldn't maintain consistent results. We are all different, and I had to learn how to tailor my vegan lifestyle to my particular needs and preferences. I learned in the process that not everything vegan is healthy for me—french fries! Five years later I have found raw vegan recipes that I *love* and can enjoy cooked vegan dishes (black-eyed peas with vegan cornbread is one of my favorites). Without trying, I have reeducated my palate such that oily, highly processed, overly cooked foods are not enjoyable, and I relish the flavor and texture of fresh foods and spices in an endless variety.

I continue to eat about 70–80 percent of my food raw for maximum nutrition, and I choose locally grown organic produce when it's available and affordable. I continue to monitor my blood pressure daily and pay attention to my body's messages as to how my last meal or stress can affect it. I engage in some form of exercise—yoga, gym, or stretching—every day. I now maintain a healthy level of readings overall without medication, as long as I eat consciously. I've even learned that I have "white coat syndrome," because my first reading in any doctor's office is typically higher. I now ask for a second or third reading, sometimes at the end of the appointment, and these are usually close to my norm.

What I did not anticipate is that as "side effects" of my plant-based eating, I would also get rid of arthritis pain, sinus congestion, my annual bout with bronchitis, and headaches.

CHAPTER 3:

How You Can Prevent or Reverse Heart Disease

"The doctor of the future will no longer treat the human frame with drugs, but rather will cure and prevent disease with nutrition."

—Thomas Edison, 1903

BECAUSE I'D EATEN A PRIMARILY vegetarian diet for many years and had no weight problem, I assumed my family's issues with hypertension and heart disease would happily pass me by. Wrong! After experiencing side effects of periodic heart palpitations and a racing heartbeat from the blood pressure medication I was prescribed, I was determined to find another solution.

I consulted a naturopathic physician who recommended that I continue my vegetarian diet with some minor changes and add herbal treatment. She also suggested a thirty-day cleanse to detox my system and jump start the healing process. One component of the cleanse was eating 80 percent raw vegetables and fruit with the option to add minimal amounts of fish or organic chicken after the first two weeks. However, I achieved only modest improvement in my hypertension.

Some months after the cleanse, she referred me to a cardiologist for a stress test and further evaluation, which ended up being one of the most interesting and life-changing doctor's visits I have ever had. Like the naturopathic physician, he took lots of time to ask questions and to talk with me. They both approached the practice of medicine as teachers as well as doctors. When he asked about my diet, I told him it was mostly vegetarian with some low-fat dairy and fish. What he said next shocked me. He explained that to reach and maintain healthy blood pressure levels, I would be much better off without the fish or dairy. I balked at first and then asked why. He said that consuming animal products produces an inflammatory response in the body that is an underlying factor in many diseases. Reading the look on my face, he went on to say that if I had to have fish, I should eat it only once or twice per month. He then assured me that the beneficial omega-3 fatty acids found in fish are available from plant sources, without the inflammation.

Finally, he said that a raw vegan diet would be the optimum way to stop the progression of my cardiovascular disease and to eliminate my hypertension. To aid the healing process, I would need to eat raw fruits and vegetables and avoid nuts and processed oils or sugars until I saw significant improvement. That's when he really lost me. He had obviously gotten similar reactions before, so he summed up the conversation by advising that I try a different thirty-day cleanse that he used with patients having a similar medical profile, during which I would eat only raw foods, no fish or chicken, and monitor my blood pressure daily. Based on the results I achieved, he would determine whether I needed to restart medication.

I left thinking "no way" to the raw diet, but I decided to try the cleanse, during which I eliminated fish. The first several days were the hardest, but by the end of the first week, it got much easier.

After the cleanse was completed, my blood pressure readings had improved enough that I was encouraged to continue feeding myself an 80–90 percent raw food diet. And in less than six months, I had given up once and for all the remaining animal protein I ate—fish, eggs, and cheese. Observing how those foods, along with cooked oils, would affect my blood pressure readings twelve to thirty-six hours later caused me to think twice before eating them. Eventually I just stopped!

I later learned that my cardiologist was one of a small but growing number of physicians treating their patients with plant-based diets as a way to gradually get them off medications. These doctors are at the forefront of "turning off the faucet, instead of mopping up the floor" by eliminating the cause of the disease as the first priority, rather than focusing on the symptoms. Using nutritional research, they have established successful diet-based programs with clinically proven results, even with very sick patients who had run out of traditional medical options.

GETTING STARTED

Since beginning my heart health recovery and vegan lifestyle, I have shared my successes with friends and family in the hope that it would open up for them new possibilities of living a healthy and joyful life free of hypertension, strokes, stents, angioplasties, bypasses, and heart attacks. I want them and all of you to know you have a choice so that you may be able to reduce, or never need to be dependent on, blood thinners (anticoagulants), ACE inhibitors, anti-platelet agents, angiotensin II receptor blockers, angiotensin-receptor inhibitors, beta blockers, calcium channel blockers, cholesterol medications, diuretics, or vasodilators—or the additional medications that are commonly prescribed for their side effects.

The first step depends on your current health status. Obviously, if you are under the care of a doctor or health care provider and taking medications for heart-related or other medical conditions, there are some things you will need to do before starting this or any other diet and lifestyle change.

1. Consult your physician and discuss your health goals. Ask for her/his support and guidance so you may safely and successfully make a dietary and lifestyle change that will help you reduce or eliminate your medications.

2. Discuss your plan, the foods you will eliminate and those you will add or increase. Physicians are becoming more open to working with their patients who want to help themselves. Ask if there are any specific foods that may interfere with any of your medications and avoid those while you are still taking those medicines, or until the doctor says they are safe. Note: Some foods like grapefruit cannot be taken with certain high blood pressure medications or other drugs.

3. Set up a follow-up visit after an agreed upon period of time to assess your status and, if necessary, make adjustments to your prescriptions.

4. Ask what steps you should take to monitor yourself (e.g. taking and tracking your daily blood pressure readings). Agree that you will call if you have any concerns.

If you are not being treated for any illness, are not taking medication, and are healthy overall, offer up your gratitude every day! You are ready to begin a journey to even better health now and especially in the years ahead. You will effectively "disease-proof" yourself not only from heart disease but also from the common diet-related illnesses of diabetes, stroke, obesity, arthritis, many cancers, and others.

FIND SUPPORT

The number one reason many people give for not making necessary food and lifestyle changes is the fear of ridicule, alienation, or of just not fitting in with friends and family. Food has a strong social component, so one of the first steps in making a positive change sustainable is to have positive people in your corner, and to surround yourself with those who will care enough not to sabotage your efforts.

Here are some tips:

1. Share what you are doing with someone you trust to support you through the ups and downs of making a life change. This could be a spouse, family member, or a friend who has demonstrated having your best interests at heart. They don't have to agree with your choice, just respect it and be your advocate when the critics sound off.
2. Spend more time with others who are making their own choices to be healthier and encourage and support them.
3. When you discuss the positive changes you are making and why, don't give people more information than they ask for, and avoid lecturing them about what they may or may not be doing for their own health. Give them the same respect regarding their choices that you want for yours. People only make changes when they are ready.
4. Don't feel that you have to defend the path you've chosen to better health. Just reaffirm that it is your choice and that you appreciate their concern.

5. To enjoy gatherings for work or with family and friends where food is served do the following: a) eat before you go so you won't be hungry and tempted to eat something you would otherwise choose not to; b) if appropriate, bring a dish that you can enjoy and share; c) when offered something you choose not to eat, I like to say, "That looks very good (if it does) but I'll pass. Thank you so much!"

6. At restaurants, you can almost always find salad or vegetable options to enjoy. Be sure to read item descriptions and ask questions about ingredients that may not be listed, particularly oils, dairy products, and meat or meat stock. If it's not a restaurant that is sensitive to those with specific food choices, eat before going so you're not hungry! I'll provide more tips on how to enjoy a healthy meal at almost any restaurant in Chapter 6.

DETOXES AND CLEANSES

Many people choose to begin a diet and lifestyle change with a period of detoxification or cleansing. This can help you reset your system by ridding it of toxin buildup. This can also give you a bit of a head start and help achieve results from your dietary change in a shorter period of time. I've found that a cleanse, detox, or period of fasting tends to disrupt eating routines or patterns you may want to move away from. They can also be a helpful first step from a psychological perspective, to set the stage for this next level of commitment to maintaining or restoring your health.

There are many detox plans and cleanses. I strongly suggest you find a natural health care practitioner, nutritionist, or health coach who will guide you to finding one that is appropriate for your needs, and who will answer any questions or concerns you may have.

WHAT DO I EAT? THE BASIC GUIDELINES

The foundation of the food plan to prevent and reverse heart disease is actually pretty simple. But when you are transitioning from the standard American diet to a vegan diet of whole vegetables, fruit, grains, legumes (beans, lentils, chickpeas, black-eyed peas, etc.), seeds, herbs, and spices, simple does not always mean easy—at least not at first.

Any lasting change requires thought and developing new habits, which is why transitions can be challenging.

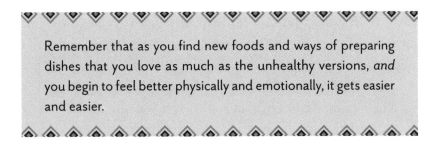

Remember that as you find new foods and ways of preparing dishes that you love as much as the unhealthy versions, *and you begin to feel better physically and emotionally*, it gets easier and easier.

There are two very similar food and lifestyle plans that have successfully reversed or improved even advanced heart disease and prevented new symptoms. The first is the result of the program and life's work of Dr. Caldwell Esselstyn Jr., beginning over forty years ago. The second is the very similar program developed by Dr. Dean Ornish, who was his contemporary. Both are based on eliminating meats and animal products from the diet, limiting fat intake, avoiding processed foods, and eating an abundance of fruit, vegetables, and other whole plant-based foods. There are some differences in the programs, which we will review so you can make a decision that fits your needs and preferences. *Both require strict adherence to achieve the results.* Once your health is restored and you are symptom free, you may make some modifications, which we will discuss at the end of this chapter.

Drs. Esselstyn and Ornish, although they've had their share of detractors within the medical establishment, each has an incredibly

> I present these two medically proven plans because they each have more than a thirty-year track record of documented success, and there were elements in each that were essential to my own reversal of heart disease symptoms.

impressive body of work, research, and growing recognition from their peers and the public as physicians.

As you might imagine, pioneering research and building a medical program that says to the public that if you eat a whole food vegan diet, you will not need drugs, stents, bypasses, and angioplasties because you will not develop heart disease, has not been well received among most physicians, or the pharmaceutical or food industries. And to further state that if you already have heart disease, and even if you have had multiple heart procedures including any or all of the above, you can actually reverse your condition and reduce or eliminate medication over time, was equally unpopular. Well, if the medical establishment didn't like that message, you can understand why they have been slow to appreciate the growing evidence that not only do programs like the Esselstyn and Ornish plans prevent or reverse heart disease, they also reverse or prevent other diet- and lifestyle-related diseases like diabetes, cancer, early stage dementia, and some auto-immune disorders. This is wonderful news for the rest of us! Let's look at an overview of both.

Dr. Caldwell Esselstyn's Plan

The Esselstyn plan is very close to the one that enabled me to reverse my hypertension and achieve a strong cardiology evaluation. The basic requirements are to:

1. Eat a plant-strong diet with a wide variety of plants including vegetables, fruit, legumes (beans, peas, lentils, of all kinds), and whole grains like oats, brown rice, wild rice, quinoa, faro, barley, whole wheat, spelt, couscous, corn, and cornmeal.

2. Eliminate *all* meat, dairy, eggs, fish, and other animal products because of their inflammatory effect on the body. Protein, omega-3 fatty acids, and all nutrients required for health and healing are abundantly available from plants. There are many delicious plant-based milks to enjoy.

3. Eliminate highly processed foods like white rice and enriched white flour, which are stripped of their nutrients and fiber and are used in most baked goods like bread, pasta, cookies, and other desserts. Most processed foods are discouraged because of added oils, sugar, salt, and preservatives; however, baked goods can be enjoyed made with whole grain flour and plant-based replacements for milk, oils, and sugar, with delicious recipes.

4. Fat is limited to 10 percent of total daily calorie intake, which is supplied in the vegetables, legumes, and grains that are make up the diet. Extracted processed oils are not used at all. That includes "healthy oils" like olive, which are really just less unhealthy, particularly for someone with heart disease.

5. Nuts are avoided altogether by those with heart disease because of their high fat content. Walnuts provide omega-3 fatty acids and may be eaten sparingly by those who do not have heart disease.

6. All fruit is included, with the caution that concentrated sugar intake from drinking fruit juices can stimulate insulin production, which can cause the liver to produce more cholesterol and lead to higher triglyceride levels. An average of three servings of fruit per day is advised. Fruit sweeteners can be consumed sparingly and used in desserts in moderate amounts.

7. Beverages include water, sparkling water (can add a little fruit juice for flavor, plant-based milks, coffee, tea, and alcohol in moderation.[12]

Since the majority of the foods you will enjoy in this plan are fresh produce, where available and affordable I prefer to buy organic or not genetically modified (non-GMO) to reduce exposure to pesticides, other chemicals, additives, and the unknown long-term effects from foods that have been genetically altered. Local fruits and vegetables are usually fresher, seasonal, and affordable. For the foods you will buy off the grocery store shelf, labels can be deceptive. Read the labels carefully because there are many loopholes in the FDA rules that manufacturers take advantage of to drive sales. "No fat" products may contain less fat overall but may still have hidden fat that will work against your health. In general, the fewer ingredients the better, and you should recognize their names.

To summarize in Dr. Esselstyn's own words, "Unlike the drugs, plant-based nutrition has beneficial effects far beyond reducing cholesterol levels. It has a mighty impact on a host of other risk factors, as well: obesity, hypertension, triglyceride, and homocysteine levels. It enables the endothelium to heal and renew itself and allows once-clogged arteries to dilate and replenish the heart muscle they serve. It makes you heart attack-proof. It doesn't get much better than that."[3]

Dr. Dean Ornish's Program

Dr. Dean Ornish's Program for Reversing Heart Disease, published in 1990, is based on a vegetarian, mostly plant-based diet as the basis for healing those with even advanced heart disease, and ensuring that those who do not have it do not get it. The foods to avoid and to enjoy are almost identical to those recommended by Dr. Caldwell Esselstyn: fruits, vegetables, whole grains, and legumes. You also avoid oils and foods with a high fat content such as nuts if you have heart disease. This diet is vegetarian and not strictly vegan because it allows egg whites and one cup of nonfat milk or yogurt per day, which are, of course, animal products, and the only ones permitted.[14]

Here are the differences in the Ornish program, which in addition to diet as the primary factor, includes more emphasis on lifestyle, stress, and emotional and spiritual aspects of the healing process.

1. Nicotine, caffeine, and alcohol are explicitly prohibited because of their influence on heart health. Advice is included on how to quit smoking.
2. Instruction is provided on the importance of exercise and how to exercise.
3. Stress management techniques are also a focus of the program including stretching, breathing, yoga, meditation, visualization techniques, and relaxation skills. Dr. Ornish also shares his own remarkable experiences in this area.
4. Social and personal relationships and improving communication and connection with the important people in our lives are also emphasized as important aspects of the healing process with counseling and professional support provided in these areas.

> On both diets you can eat an abundance of the allowed foods, and virtually all you want of most of them, and still regain your health while losing weight without any extra effort.

The stories told by participants in both the Esselstyn and Ornish heart disease reversal programs are moving and compelling. Not only would many of them not be alive without the knowledge and support they received, most experienced other unexpected health benefits, as well as significant improvements in their quality and enjoyment of life.[15]

The plan introduced to me by my cardiologist is very similar to the Esselstyn program in that it is totally plant-based with no exceptions. During the healing process, it also restricts all oils, nuts, and highly processed foods, but goes a step further to prescribe 100 percent raw foods. I have modified my maintenance diet to add back some cooked foods I enjoy like beans with brown rice, cornbread with black-eyed peas, baked sweet potatoes, Brussels sprouts (which are super high in omega-3 fatty acids, especially when cooked), and many others. Now I can eat raw nuts like walnuts and almonds sparingly because unprocessed they are a good source of healthy fat. I am mindful not eat so many of them that I increase my daily fat intake from all sources above 10–15 percent. Avocados are another favorite whole food to provide healthy fat. *The point is to eat the whole food in moderation and not the extracted oils.* I have shared some of my favorite dishes in the recipe section of this book. I still eat what I describe as a "high raw" vegan diet, keeping the percentage of raw foods around 70–80 percent. This is now for me a preference as much as a health choice because I love the colors, flavors, and textures of vegetables just as they are when harvested.

It is also true that cooking can destroy beneficial enzymes in food that enable the body to utilize many of the nutrients they contain. For those reasons, a high raw diet works for me, and in addition, I have met many talented raw vegan chefs whose dishes will make you forget about the cooked versions!

My daily meditation, yoga, and two or three weekly trips to my local YMCA for a thirty-to forty-five-minute cardio workout are more aligned with the emphasis on these kinds of activities in the Ornish program. I find immense value in them and highly recommend including stress relief, mindfulness, and physical activities of your choice in your healing or stay-healthy plan. These for me are indispensable components of whole self-care and the joy and fulfillment that it brings.

HOW TO CHOOSE AND PERSONALIZE YOUR PLAN

The data and science are clear that a plant-based diet provides a baseline for preventing and reversing heart disease and other Western life-style diseases like hypertension, diabetes, cancer, obesity, and dementia. Eating and caring for your body in the manner described above will help you prevent or reverse these illnesses and more. It leads to a healthy, more balanced life full of joy and appreciation for the simple things—food, relationships, a connection to nature, and the awareness that we are part of an endless cycle of life and its regeneration.

I credit my healing process to aspects of both of these programs with a couple of modifications that I found both appealing and helpful.

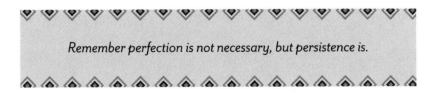

Remember perfection is not necessary, but persistence is.

Change is difficult at first and persisting through the stumbles on our way to a healthier life is part of the journey. The state of our health when beginning our food journey will determine the minimum we must do to achieve results and will impact the amount of time our healing takes. Again, persistence is the key while our new healthier habits are forming.

My diagnoses seven years ago included hypertension, an enlarged heart, and arteriosclerosis (artery hardening). I did not have advanced heart disease (no stents, angioplasties, bypasses, or heart attacks). However, because of my family history, my cardiologist's diagnosis, and my own research on heart disease and its progression, I made the decision to commit to an exclusively plant-based diet and eliminate all animal foods. There were other factors in this decision that have to do with the conditions under which food animals live and are slaughtered, the focus of big agriculture and big drug companies on profits rather than health or ethics, and my belief that we are one with our natural environment. Human health suffers when we lose our connection to and appreciation for the environment that sustains us and our compassion for ourselves and others. These aspects of my food and lifestyle choices are a thread running through this book, and I will discuss them more fully in its conclusion.

In summary, here is the plan I still follow:
1. A detox cleanse was part of my initial introduction to eating to reverse high blood pressure and other heart disease symptoms, and periodically I have done others. However, the better I eat, the less frequently I feel the need to detox.
2. A strictly vegan diet, with the exception of raw organic honey, which I choose for its health benefits and taste;

preference, not a requirement, for organic and non-genetically modified foods where available and affordable; local food sources preferred, including small local farmers.

3. Seventy to eighty percent raw food for optimum nutrition, and the ability to absorb and utilize it. I also prefer the taste and bright colors of raw food, both of which are diminished in the heat of cooking. The diminished taste and texture from cooking is often offset by adding fat, salt, or sugar.

4. All the vegetables and fruit I want; brown rice, whole grains, black beans, pinto beans, garbanzo beans, lentils, and black-eyed peas, to name a few; lots of spices and herbs.

5. Sprouted whole-grain breads, and cereals.

6. Grain and seed milks (favorites are hempseed and oat milk), which may have less fat than nut milks.

7. Dates, fruit juice, and maple syrup for sweeteners, in addition to raw honey.

8. Avoidance of mainstream packaged or processed foods because of chemical additives, colors, preservatives, and long lists of ingredients I cannot recognize or pronounce.

9. Preference for meals I prepare at home. I save money, the ingredients are fresh, and I know what they are.

10. Avoidance of processed oils (including olive oil) in meals, cooking, or salads. Keep fat intake to 10–15 percent of total daily diet by limiting nuts, nut butters, and foods with high saturated fat content like coconut spreads and butters.

11. Supplements for vitamin B-12 and vitamin D; glucosamine and turmeric supplements for joint health and their antioxidant benefit, especially protecting the body against oxidative stress from environmental pollutants and other substances that play a role in aging and disease.

12. Support of vegan and health-conscious restaurants and food stores for the quality of their products. It is vital to

keep them strong and to keep the availability for healthy food for everyone growing!

13. Daily yoga and meditation; minimum forty-five minutes of cardio two or three times per week.

For the first time in my life, I enjoy preparing meals. The variety of vegetables, fruit, grains, legumes, spices, and herbs I now consume, and the many recipes and choices for cooking, baking, or preparing them inspire me to be creative and try new things. I love to eat, enjoy, and celebrate great food! In the following chapters we will explore some exciting new food options, recipes, and herbs and spices to make your healthy food journey a source of daily pleasure and adventure.

CHAPTER 4:

Overcoming Food Addictions and Cravings

"In order not to abuse food I have to stay fully conscious and aware of every bite, of taking time and chewing slowly. I have to focus on being fully alive, awake, present and engaged, connected in every area of my life."

—OPRAH WINFREY, 2009

ADDICTIONS OF ALL TYPES ARE perhaps more common than we would like to admit. We certainly know the dangers of drug, alcohol, and other substance abuse. However, addiction to food can be just as devastating to long-term health and vitality, even though it may not carry the same social stigma. In the extreme, there are those who binge on certain foods or use food as a coping mechanism to deal with the stresses in their lives. More common, however, are the food cravings that most of us experience at one point or another. Desire for sugar-filled, fatty, and highly processed foods can seem overpowering, even when the health risks are clearly understood.

SUGAR ADDICTION

In a *New York Times* article on the "science" of addictive junk food, author Michael Moss talked about how food companies "pretty much ignore health and nutrition in order to get more people to buy and eat their products. Sugar and fat are the leading 'go to' additives for the food industry to give food that addictive quality."[16]

There is a reason we find it hard to resist fat-rich, sweet foods. Sugar is one of the most powerfully addictive substances going back to the beginning of human history. Early primates, including man, ate a diet consisting mainly of plants. And of the plant sources available, fruits were rare compared to edible grasses and vegetables. Because sugar gave fruits higher calorie content, our ancestors who ate them had an advantage against starvation, increased their chance of survival, and had the opportunity to pass on their gene pool. The sugar in fruits was very healthy for earliest man, because of the small amounts available to him.

A 2012 *New York Times* article by Harvard professor Daniel Lieberman entitled "Evolution's Sweet Tooth" states that "For millions of years, our cravings and digestive systems were exquisitely balanced because sugar was rare. Apart from honey, most of the foods our hunter-gatherer ancestors ate were no sweeter than a carrot. The invention of farming made starchy foods more abundant, but it wasn't until very recently that technology made pure sugar bountiful. The food industry has made a fortune because we retain Stone Age bodies that crave sugar but live in a Space Age world in which sugar is cheap and plentiful.[17] Scientists have found that high consumption of processed sugar (sucrose) and high-fructose corn syrup leads to behavioral and neurochemical changes much like those seen in substance abuse. *Sugar stimulates the same pleasure centers as cocaine and heroin.* They have validated what we see around us or may have experienced at times ourselves: sugar leads to cravings and is highly addictive.

FLOUR ADDICTION

In addition to sugar, flour addiction is surprisingly common. White flour is stripped of its wheat kernel, which makes it super easy for our digestive system to convert it into glucose or sugar. Be aware that many whole wheat bread products are also made with white flour, with coloring and wheat bran added for appearance and texture, so they're actually not that different from white bread from a health standpoint. Again, read the label! Modern steel milling turns the wheat kernel into a white powdery substance that is dangerously stripped of nutritional value. Manufacturers then add man-made replicas of nutrients, which are not the equivalent of those found in whole foods, to give it some food value. The benefit to the food industry is that the result is a product that has an incredibly long shelf life and is pest resistant, probably because little remains in it that pests are interested in.

New hybrid species of wheat introduced in the last fifty or sixty years produce bigger yields, and have a higher concentration of gluten, which gives products made with it more elasticity and makes them fluffier. It may be one of the reasons why Celiac disease was largely unknown until the latter part of the twentieth century.

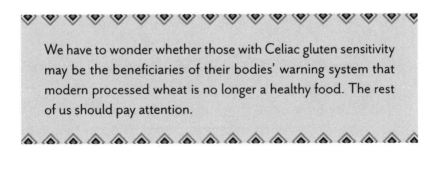

We have to wonder whether those with Celiac gluten sensitivity may be the beneficiaries of their bodies' warning system that modern processed wheat is no longer a healthy food. The rest of us should pay attention.

According to Dr. Mark Hyman, author of *The Blood Sugar Solution*, "This new modern wheat may look like wheat, but it is different in three important ways that all drive obesity, diabetes, heart disease, cancer, dementia, and more. It contains a super starch, amylopectin A, that is super fattening, a form of super gluten that is super inflammatory, and [acts like] a super drug that is super addictive and makes you crave and eat more."[18]

FORMING HEALTHY FOOD HABITS—
A SIMPLE SECRET

How do we overcome sugar, flour, and other food cravings or addictions? In the case of addiction, "kicking the habit" initially requires some type of intervention, or detoxification period, usually accompanied by symptoms of withdrawal. Because food addictions and poor dietary habits are so common, there are many detox programs, diets, and cleanses on the market designed for this purpose. If you feel you may have a food addiction, I recommend seeking the advice of a health care professional in choosing a detox program that is appropriate and safe for your needs, and who will offer support and counseling during and after the process. Food addiction, like most addictive behavior, is known to have a psychological component. It often involves eating to cope with or compensate for feelings of loss, fear, anxiety, depression, or unworthiness. This is the reason for the inclusion of psychological counseling and group therapy in the Dean Ornish program outlined earlier. If you believe you have a food addiction, there are resources to help, starting with your personal physician or health care organization. Resources can also be found at http://foodaddictionresearch.org/resources.[19]

The problem for all of us is, how do we maintain and build upon the results once we have taken the first steps toward a healthier lifestyle and better eating habits? How do we incorporate the healthy aspects that we are learning, and how do we form new eating and self-care habits that will maintain and further improve the healthy new start? Some years ago, I attended a seminar where a motivational speaker said something that has stuck with me because of its simple truth. His topic was how to make positive change and break negative habits. "Don'ts don't work" was the basis of his advice. The more we focus on what it is that we do *not* want to do, the more irresistible it becomes. He challenged us to try it. "Don't look at my tie," he said from the podium. Of course, from that moment, it was impossible not to sneak a peek.

He went on to explain that to successfully break a habit, you have to focus on forming the new one you want to replace it. This is simple genius. Perhaps you've noticed that when people go on a "diet" they always talk about what they can't eat. And when they come off the diet these are the first things they can't wait to devour! This is why traditional diets never work. If someone succeeds in achieving weight loss or other health goals by traditional dieting, it is because somewhere in the process they develop the habit of eating in a healthier way that is also physically and psychologically satisfying. It's not the diet that works, it's the formation of a new habit or set of habits that can create lasting results.

The "don'ts don't work" principle is true for people with health problems who can also quickly recite all the foods the doctor has said they can't have. You can feel the sense of loss and longing, even if they don't come right out and say how much they miss eating them. The truth is that they have not found new food choices that they have learned to love as much the ones that made them sick. Sadly, most people don't even know this is possible. It is the reason why plans presented in Chapter 3 for preventing and reversing heart disease and other diet-related diseases focus on healthy and delicious alternatives to the foods that contribute to the illnesses. We need to focus on where we are going and how to make the journey enjoyable!

Dr. Susan Thompson, author of *Bright Line Eating*, is an expert on food addiction and a recovering addict herself who battled obesity as a child and young adult. Although "don'ts don't work," when something definitely unhealthy for us seems also irresistible, we need clear boundaries or a clear bright line that we don't cross, to give ourselves a way out. Most of us seeking to reverse lifestyle diseases by changing how and what we eat will probably battle with food cravings more than food addiction. Nevertheless, to actually reverse disease, adherence to the plan we commit to is required, including the foods to avoid during the healing process. So, no meat means no meat, not meat only on Sunday. And no dairy means no dairy, not a little bit in our coffee. *Only after the disease is no longer present and our health status changes as a result can we consider reintroducing any of the eliminated foods that can be beneficial for a healthy adult.* Typically, after experiencing the difference in how we feel, energy levels, and outlook on life, and having found so many great-tasting healthy foods to enjoy without worry, a growing number of us find their way to make the new habits a permanent part of their lifestyle.

I mentioned earlier that my healthy eating journey has evolved over three decades in mostly small steps. I drew my own "bright lines" around certain foods or methods of food preparation as I grew more aware of my body's reaction to them and sought out information to understand why they no longer served me. At the same time, I experimented with healthier foods or methods of preparation that made me feel better when I ate them. One of my first bright lines was drawn around certain fried foods, initially as a reaction to how I felt after eating a drive-thru lunch of fried chicken and french fries, for example. Eventually I eliminated all fried foods, which happened naturally over the years as my taste and preference for them faded. Taste and preference are mostly determined by what we are accustomed to, and as we develop new preferences, we start to gravitate toward them while the old ones gradually lose much of their appeal. I remember many years ago switching from whole milk to low fat. A few months later I had house guests and bought some whole milk for them. After they left, I tried some of the milk on cereal and literally had trouble eating it. It was hard to believe that my preference had changed so dramatically so quickly, and it taught me a valuable lesson about change. Now oat and other seed milks are just as satisfying!

At other times, my version of a bright line was drawn around a single type of food or beverage. One of those was soda. I gave up the sugared, artificially flavored ones in favor of the artificially sweetened and flavored ones, and then gave them all up. One of the things I discovered that tasted much better and was healthier by comparison was adding a little fresh fruit juice to sparkling water to make a "natural" sparkling drink with no refined sugar or artificial sweetener. Ultimately it wasn't the "don't drink sodas" that worked but rather taking the first steps toward finding a more satisfying and enjoyable alternative.

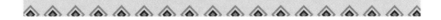

Although I eliminated most meats over time—first pork, then beef, then chicken, and finally fish, followed by dairy and eggs—my bright line moment in which I once and for all chose an all-plant-based diet came more than twenty years later, while watching an interview with former NBA player John Salley, in which he said he would no longer eat anything that had a heart or a face. With the health benefits having long been demonstrated, at that moment it was his simple statement advocating the humane treatment of animals and ending needless slaughter and abuse that made my decision final, and easy. Having found plant-based foods that I loved allowed me to maintain it.

MOVING FORWARD

Once we understand that our potential for health and happiness is only limited by the choices we make, the path forward with options and support for our goals starts to reveal itself. In our new awareness or mindfulness, rather than fighting against our bad habits and poor choices, we begin a journey of discovering new passions, new delights, and healthier ways of living, including the pure joy of eating well. This includes foods that are colorful, delicious, and either simple or sophisticated in their preparation, presentation, and flavor combinations. Through the combination of spices, textures, and flavors of whole and minimally processed foods, any traditional culinary experience can be recreated as a healthy alternative choice. We can have it all—naturally and in abundance!

Instead of quietly craving that serving of fries every time we pass a McDonald's billboard, we can admit that we like the taste and the texture, and then say yes to a generous serving of baked sweet potato sticks for dinner or make sweet potato chips in the oven. Craving a hamburger? Just Google veggie burger online, and you will find an endless number of recipes for vegetable-based, high-protein burger patties, made from portabella, falafel, black beans, and other vegetables, with an equally wide variety of spices and natural flavors for great taste. Do you like mustard? There are a number of organic, all-natural choices on the market, or you can make you own fresh and customized to your taste. Nothing has to be missed in the taste category while you take steps toward good health in your own food adventure.

I know what you're thinking. What about dessert? For those of us who can enjoy sweet treats, how about a creamy hemp milkshake that you can make in minutes, sweetened with dates? And one of my favorite treats is a recipe for Rip's Oatmeal Raisin Chocolate Chip Cookies that I found online that only takes twenty minutes from start to finish. Find it in *The Engine 2 Cookbook* by Rip Esselstyn, one of several heart-healthy cookbooks, found in the Resources section. And a fruit smoothie is always a satisfying and healthy sweet treat. These are not necessarily "low fat" or "low sugar" foods but they can be made healthier with our choice of ingredients. They are treats, and healthy because they satisfy the body's nutritional needs by providing beneficial proteins and nutrients along *with* their calories. And just as importantly, when I choose to eat them, I take the time to really enjoy them without guilt, which is also healthy. And I eat less because they are delicious and satisfying. As I have gradually moved my food choices to more whole and raw organic foods, I find that I look forward to these and other healthier treats and am less and less tempted by the traditional, not so healthy ones.

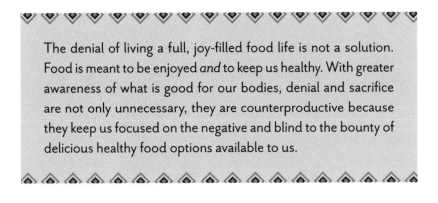

The denial of living a full, joy-filled food life is not a solution. Food is meant to be enjoyed *and* to keep us healthy. With greater awareness of what is good for our bodies, denial and sacrifice are not only unnecessary, they are counterproductive because they keep us focused on the negative and blind to the bounty of delicious healthy food options available to us.

The awareness that we are beings with unlimited potential in an abundant universe is a mind shift that changes the way we view ourselves, and the world around us. *In food as in life, find what you love and what loves you back, and go for it!* I will focus the following chapters on how to do just that.

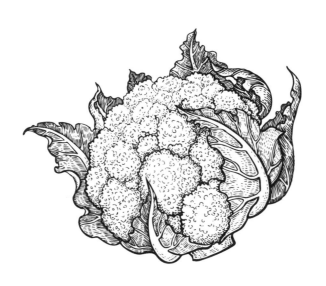

CHAPTER 5:

Reclaiming the Joy of Eating

"If you truly get in touch with a piece of carrot, you get in touch with the soil, the rain, the sunshine. You get in touch with Mother Earth and eating in such a way, you feel in touch with true life, your roots, and that is meditation. If we chew every morsel of our food in that way, we become grateful, and when you are grateful, you are happy."
—THICH NHAT HANH, spiritual leader and peace activist

WE ALL HAVE TO EAT TO LIVE, and almost everyone enjoys the pleasure of favorite foods. These tend to be foods we learned to enjoy as children and are often associated with fond memories. I will always remember my first bakery shop birthday cake! It was not only the sweetest of confections, it literally melted in my mouth and was so pretty with its pink roses, green leaves, and my name spelled out in beautiful lavender strokes. In the 1950s no one, or at least no one I knew, was in the least bit worried about the health impact of refined sugar, let alone refined, bleached flour. Sugar was only an issue for diabetics, and that disease was uncommon compared to the epidemic levels we see today. My mother's only concern was that I didn't eat so much that I would rot my teeth.

I also loved chocolate and still do. Our Friday family night out usually involved a trip to the local Dairy Queen for burgers, hot dogs, fries, and of course, a chocolate milkshake for me. Life was good, and I continued to love these and similar foods well into adulthood, until my body started to object. At first I thought the lower energy levels and extra pounds were the result of "normal" aging. Unfortunately, they are still "normal" today for someone with my food and lifestyle choices at the time. Although making healthier food choices flies in the face of the standard American diet with its images of birthday cake and ice cream, Thanksgiving turkey, Fourth of July barbecues, and hotdogs with fries at the ballpark, the changes in my body prompted my interest in learning what I could do to feel better and regain my energy.

This was the beginning of my commitment to take care of my body, maintain a healthy weight, and avoid deteriorating health.

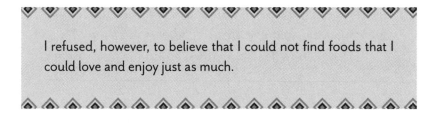

I refused, however, to believe that I could not find foods that I could love and enjoy just as much.

Avoiding weight gain is what most people think of as the primary reason for eating healthier, mostly driven by a "thin is beautiful" standard. As a result, we spend millions annually for weight-loss diets, pills, herbs, instant wraps, surgery, and more to achieve the image, often at the risk of our health. In American culture, we have this conflicted relationship with food. There is a new fad diet every month, it seems, and despite the fact that Americans spend over $60 billion annually to lose weight, obesity is on the rise along with the serious health issues that go with it.

We focus so much on the exterior, we miss the point that health and beauty come from the inside out. By focusing on fad weight loss products and treatments, we divert our attention and resources away from healthy and sustainable food and lifestyle choices, while our underlying health actually declines. The overwhelming amount of advertising information and disinformation aimed at selling a pill, procedure, or cosmetic quick fix sets us up for failure after failure to achieve and sustain results and ensures a ready market for the next fad.

The bad news is there are no quick fixes for health conditions that are the result of years of poor choices. The good news is that each of us has the power to change our health and our lives for the better one good choice after another, day by day, and it's never too late to start. By making my own choice to do just that, I have found people and resources, often in unexpected places, ready to support and guide me, and so will you: it's a principle of natural law. Whatever we endeavor to achieve, the universe has a way of orchestrating events, people, and circumstances to support the fulfillment of our intent. Everything we need to be successful is accessible to us when we are ready, and we simply ask.

BEAUTY, SIMPLICITY, AND ABUNDANCE

One of the unexpected benefits of reclaiming our health, and the joy of feeding ourselves mindfully, is the greater appreciation of simple, natural whole foods just as they are when harvested.

I look forward to those moments, sometimes unexpected, when an orange is so sweet, so juicy, and with just the right amount of tartness that I stop and give thanks while I savor a bite. Or when an ear of corn is perfectly crunchy with its own sweet finish eaten right off the cob.

And how I love a salad of baby kale mixed with deep green, pungent arugula that reminds me of the tang of the fresh mustard greens I grew up eating in Texas, but with a fresher taste, unaltered by cooking. I love these tastes and textures; however, the appreciation of these foods is enhanced by the very process of eating them consciously, with gratitude for their enjoyment combined with an understanding of their healing properties.

Good health starts with our grocery lists and making sure they contain a wide variety of whole fresh fruits, vegetables, legumes, grains, and other unprocessed foods. Now that I know it is absolutely possible to avoid the heart disease, Alzheimer's, and diabetes so common in my family, this is important to me. I am drawn to the wisdom of Hippocrates, the father of modern medicine, who said in 430 BC, "Let food be thy medicine and medicine be thy food." With this in mind, I include some specific foods on my grocery list that are known to help fight inflammation and boost my immune system, including garlic, celery, basil, walnuts, and grapefruit. See the list of seasonal foods with healing properties on pages 64–65. In general, any fresh fruit, vegetable, nut, or grain will have in its whole, unprocessed state, many health benefits to offer. And eating a wide variety of whole foods is even more beneficial, because each has something unique that our bodies need, and all are made more effective when they are part of a varied diet. Combining a wide variety of foods and spices in delicious recipes feeds our senses and our souls as well as our bodies.

The next step is a visit to my grocer's fresh produce section or a trip to a local farmers' market or farm co-op. I look for organic items where available and affordable, non-GMO, in season, and local fruits and vegetables. The Environmental Working Group (EWG) is an independent watchdog, research, and information source on food safety and related environmental issues. On their website https://www.ewg.org/foodnews, they publish annual lists of foods that they call the "Dirty Dozen" and "Clean Fifteen," based on the amount of pesticide residues they contain.[20]

I try to limit foods that have traveled from other regions of the world, but when I do buy them, I look for "fair trade" certified, sustainably produced foods to ensure, to the extent that I can, that I am supporting farmers and companies that are good Earth stewards. For staples like spices, sweeteners, whole grain flours, or plant-based milks, I look for those that are organic, non-GMO, and have ingredients I recognize. If you want juices, look for cold-pressed ones in the refrigerated section that are alive with enzymes and probiotic properties that have not been destroyed by heat. Remember that extracted fruit juices contain relatively high concentrations of sugars in the form of fructose, glucose, and sucrose. This will likely be a problem for those who have or are concerned about diabetes. Also remember that too much sugar can trigger an increase in triglycerides which affects heart health, so we all should be aware. I've made the decision not to drink sweet juices like apple, orange, and pineapple, and instead to eat the whole fruit or use it in smoothies, to avoid sugar spikes and the danger of feeding insulin resistance. Eating the whole fruit with its fiber is how nature intended us to enjoy the juice.

Finally, I always look for something new and seasonal to try—a different green leafy vegetable, a fruit I don't often eat, a different grain or spice, or just a new variety of apple. We live in an amazingly abundant universe. There are more than twenty thousand species of edible plants, grains, nuts, and seeds on planet Earth that provide everything our bodies require nutritionally. They naturally contain the properties to support perfect health and wellness, as well as remedies for illness when our health is compromised. However, approximately twenty species make up 90 percent of our diet. There are so many other choices out there to explore.

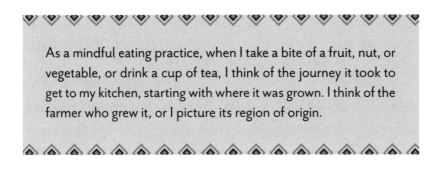

As a mindful eating practice, when I take a bite of a fruit, nut, or vegetable, or drink a cup of tea, I think of the journey it took to get to my kitchen, starting with where it was grown. I think of the farmer who grew it, or I picture its region of origin.

I often think of a food's history and evolution into the particular variety or form I am enjoying. I sometimes think it would be interesting to research those journeys, although I have not as yet done that. It is humbling and fascinating just to contemplate all the events over hundreds or thousands of years that led to the exact food that I now have the privilege of enjoying.

EATING A PERSIMMON IN FALL

Last September I saw a beautiful display of reddish-orange persimmons at the supermarket. It immediately reminded me of the ones that grew wild in East Texas. I particularly remember the little stand of persimmon trees along the five-minute walk from my house to my grandmother's. I thought about the ones I ate too early before they reached the soft, sweet, juicy-ripe state and how they drew my mouth and lips into a tight pucker. And then I remembered how perfectly sweet and good they were when eaten at just the right time, so I bought one.

Every other day or so, I would gently press my finger against this persimmon to test its ripeness. I did not want to eat it too soon, or too late, when the flesh would be too soft or mushy. This went on for two or three weeks, and I started to feel like I'd made a bad choice, and that it would never be just right. At least it looked striking sitting on top of the other fruit and a couple of acorn squash in my basket on the kitchen counter. One morning it felt just a little bit softer to the touch, and I decided this was it! I rinsed and carefully removed the skin. I cut off the stem on the flower side and then sliced it into four or five round slices with perfect star shapes at the center of each, so pretty and unique beside the blueberries, blackberries, sliced watermelon, oranges, and pears on my breakfast plate.

After this long and patient courtship with my persimmon, I took the first bite. Oh, my God, was it worth the wait! It had a clean, pure, sweet flavor and perfect texture. It made my ground raw flax and pumpkin seed "cereal" sing when I took a bite of one and chased it with the other. It was the first and last thing I ate that morning, because I wanted the pleasure to last as long as possible. I found out later from my daughter that this was not the same variety of persimmon that grew wild in Texas, and I could have eaten it while it was firm. I'm sort of glad I didn't know.

When I thought of possible titles for this little book, I was attracted to the concept of joy because of experiences like this one. Love, patience, timing—mine and infinitely more so, Earth's, with its cycle of life—created the ecstatic and pleasurable experience of eating this simple food, in its natural state, just as it came from the ground.

◇◇◇◇◇◇◇◇◇◇◇◇

The fact that I could have this experience with something that is absolutely good for me, with joy and no guilt, is extraordinarily humbling. This beautiful little persimmon had not been put into any chef's dish on the menu in a fancy restaurant. It was not sugared, pureed, caramelized, baked, or juiced. To have done anything other than to eat it just as it was in that moment would have been a missed opportunity. It was sheer perfection and needed no help to be so.

The foods we need to nourish joyful, healthy, and happy lives are available to us naturally, from Earth, and in great abundance and variety. They are a product of its intelligence, as we are, along with every living being, cloud, or river. We make life more complicated than it needs to be and, by choice, we can return to the simple things to reclaim and relish what is important. It is fine to have all the popular comforts, conveniences, and "stuff" that we are conditioned to value and to strive for. But do these things lead us to happiness, health, and fulfillment? We may want those things, but to believe that we must have them to be happy is an entirely different matter. Food is one of our most fundamental needs. Healthy food and a healthy environment are our right, and the stewardship of Earth, which produces both, is our responsibility.

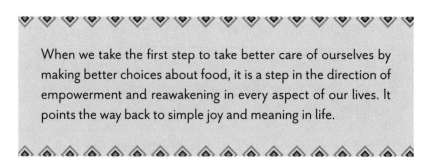

When we take the first step to take better care of ourselves by making better choices about food, it is a step in the direction of empowerment and reawakening in every aspect of our lives. It points the way back to simple joy and meaning in life.

SLOW FOOD—PATIENCE AND APPRECIATION

Enjoying and eating food mindfully starts with appreciating the health we do have, and Earth that provides in abundance everything we need to enhance and nourish it. We have to stop and taste the persimmon.

Feeding ourselves consciously takes time and patience at first, like anything new. We live in a fast-paced, convenience-oriented society. We like high-speed technology, instant gratification, and fast food. Why do we never seem to have enough time for the things we say we value, including family, friends, and our quality of life? Some would say that we live much of our lives unconsciously. We are creatures of routine and habit. We wake up, grab a quick coffee and pastry as we head off to work, get a sandwich and soft drink for lunch, and are so tired by the time we get home at the end of the day that we default to processed convenience foods from a package. We color inside the lines even when we've forgotten why.

It is our human nature to try to fit in, to do and act like those around us. We want to believe that if we do so, we will lead happy, healthy, and productive lives, and that our society is set up to safeguard our right to do so. Well it is and it isn't. We do have the right to expect our health care system to work, our food supply to be safe, and our educational institutions to prepare us to think critically and to use our knowledge in ways that make our communities and the world a better place for our children to grow up in.

However, our society also safeguards a free market economy, and the right of corporations and the business community to make a profit by bringing products to market that we are free to buy or not buy. There are certainly regulations in place that in most cases prevent egregious and obviously dangerous practices. However, as we see in the news every day, there is a lot of gray area . . . like abusive factory animal farming, the marketing of unlabeled genetically modified foods, and widespread use of cancer-causing pesticides, just to name a few.

When it comes to our health and how we feed and take care of ourselves and our families, we will not have all of the answers. Companies spend hundreds of millions of advertising and marketing dollars to make their products appealing by using buzz words like "lite," "natural," and "healthy." They emphasize what they know we as consumers want to hear and are silent about what they know to be potential health issues.

The Latin phrase *caveat emptor* which translates to "let the buyer beware" basically means it is our responsibility to inform ourselves and protect our own best interests, even when we are buying food. Fewer ingredients are better, and definitely avoid those with long complicated names that sound like they belong in a laboratory, because that's probably where they came from.

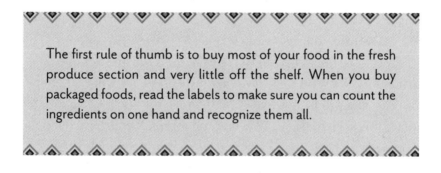

The first rule of thumb is to buy most of your food in the fresh produce section and very little off the shelf. When you buy packaged foods, read the labels to make sure you can count the ingredients on one hand and recognize them all.

RECREATING FOOD TRADITIONS

There is nothing wrong with honoring our food traditions by eating the foods our parents and grandparents ate, as long as we make conscious choices about how to eat them and how much. We first need to choose fruits, grains, and vegetables that are organically grown when affordable, and therefore pesticide free and sustainably produced. That was not an issue when our grandparents grew their own food on family farms, when the fertilizer came from the cow pen, and "farm-to-table" was more than a slogan. And if we choose to eat meat or fish, we should look for labels to certify that the animals are treated ethically and produced in a manner that does not contaminate or harm the environment. The meat or fish may cost a little more because of the quality, but if you eat it less often, you will save money overall and enjoy better health. Remember that a few decades ago, having meat at every meal was considered a luxury, and we were healthier because of it. You will save the difference at the doctor's office and the pharmacy many times over.

In addition to our own favorites, there is a world of food possibilities based on the culinary traditions of other cultures. In the next chapters we will explore other cuisines and how they can add to our healthy and delicious options. When we open our minds and hearts to new experiences, and use our creativity and imagination, there are unlimited possibilities to prepare and enjoy food we will simply love . . . and that will love us back! Now that is good food karma!

part 2:
sh🍓pping and
healthy food
options

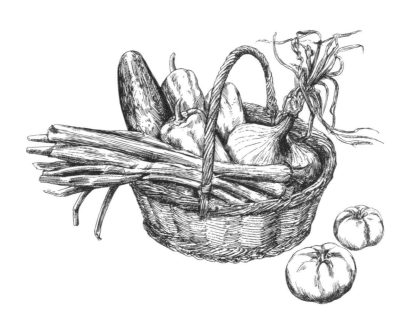

CHAPTER 6:

Fruits and Veggies: Eat All You Want!

"If you keep good food in your fridge, you will eat good food."

—Erik McAdams, health and fitness coach

THE BEST THING ABOUT WHOLE FRUITS and vegetables, in addition to disease-proofing us from systemic inflammation and chronic health issues, is that you can eat all you want! They are particularly beneficial when you eat them raw, in salads or smoothies in infinite combinations, or in recipes with minimal cooking. The delicious recipes featured in this book will require minimum prep and cooking times, so you have more time to enjoy them. The nutritional power of fruits and vegetables lies not only in their vitamins, minerals, and protein. Just as importantly, it is in their enzymes, which uncooked, can best deliver many nutrients to the body in a form it can use. When eaten in variety, they can arguably sustain life and vitality on their own. Adding nuts, seeds, legumes, and grains provides all our nutritional requirements along with a limitless variety of preparation methods and taste and texture sensations.

SHOPPING TIPS: LOCAL AND SEASONAL

The freshest, most nutritious fruits and vegetables are the ones that are not shipped from halfway around the world before they arrive on your table. The concept of living mindfully means that our choices are made in awareness of the impact on our own individual health and enjoyment, along with the health of our communities and our environment. By supporting local farmers, we help reduce the environmental impact and cost of transporting food over long distances. Local family farms tend to be smaller producers, and by buying from them, we support our local communities. Choose those who demonstrate that they avoid chemicals and pesticides in favor of organic and Earth-friendly fertilizers and pest control methods, even if they are not certified organic. "Know your farmer, know your food" is more than a slogan; it is another way to protect your health and invest in farmers who are trying to do it right. It's also a very important opportunity to reconnect with nature and experience thankfulness for the natural abundance around us.

My visits to Finca Tres Robles urban farm, and other farms in my local area, have been lessons in gratitude. First, I was humbled by the amount of physical labor required on the part of the farmers and volunteers to produce the food that most of us take for granted, and the care and commitment that was evident among them. The second lesson in appreciation was the way that things our society throws away—wood chips, coffee grounds, vegetable scraps—are used by organic and sustainable farms to increase the quality and yield of their crops without chemicals, making their operations highly efficient. The third eye-opener was the diversity of the crops produced. In addition to kale, collards, onions, tomatoes, squash, okra, and other local favorites, there were always some delicious new varieties of vegetables or fruits to try, all fresh from the garden.

I've now tried fresh moringa, African basil, Persian eggplant, and edible hibiscus leaves, which have a fresh lemony taste. The cultivation of many different kinds of plants, known as biodiversity, helps protect and enrich the soil and also provides the kind of variety in our diets that is known to improve our health.

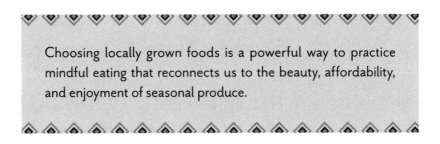

Choosing locally grown foods is a powerful way to practice mindful eating that reconnects us to the beauty, affordability, and enjoyment of seasonal produce.

These foods arrive fresh to local markets and, because of lower transportation costs and seasonal abundance, they are great nutritional and budget-friendly choices. Because they are fresh and in season, their quality, flavor, and variety offer big pluses for delighting the taste buds and the wallet. As a bonus, the variety makes it easy to add a new twist to favorite recipes.

By making local, seasonal produce the staple of our diet, we naturally build variety into our daily meals. Eating these foods also ties us to Earth's natural cycles with foods whose properties will help our bodies adapt to seasonal weather changes in the areas in which we live.

Spring

Depending on where we live, in spring we can enjoy fresh local strawberries, grapefruit, tomatoes, onions, celery, cauliflower, carrots, cabbage, beets, broccoli, and so much more. Spring vegetables like asparagus and artichokes are also allergy fighters. Mustard greens, a favorite in the American South, have glucosinolates, which fight cancer and inflammation and, when cooked or steamed, may help lower cholesterol. Arugula, carrots, radishes, green peas, and Swiss chard are other springtime favorites that are nutrient rich and have antioxidants and many other health benefits. Swiss Chard, for example, is rich in vitamin K and nitrates, which can help lower blood pressure and improve circulation, making it particularly heart healthy. These foods are less likely to trigger inflammation, an underlying source of spring seasonal allergies.

Summer

There is an abundance of blackberries, cucumbers, squash, turnips, corn, mushrooms, peaches, watermelon, cantaloupe, nectarines, pears, potatoes, blueberries, and apples in summer gardens and orchards. These summer fruits have a high water content, which helps us maintain hydration on hot summer days. Summer fruits and vegetables also have a high content of vitamins C and E, which help protect the skin from sun damage.

Fall

In fall there are apples, cabbage, carrots, cucumbers, potatoes, squash, collards, Swiss chard, kale, onions, pumpkins, pecans, and dates. An article published by Rachel Metzer Warren entitled "Seasonal Eating for Your Body," states that "Foods rich in quercetin, an antioxidant in onions, grapes, and apples, may reduce susceptibility to the flu virus. And foods that contain the antioxidant allicin—such as garlic, onions, and chives—also pack antiviral properties. Just be sure to crush garlic and let it sit for five minutes or so before using, or chop and eat raw in a salad to maximize its disease-fighting potential."[21]

Winter

In winter there are oranges, lemons, grapefruit, beets, broccoli, cabbage, collard and mustard greens, tomatoes, squash, pomegran-ates, and cranberries. We have a tendency in winter to eat lots of carbohydrates as we enjoy comfort foods to warm us and lift our spirits. Unfortunately, this can also add unwanted pounds because we are generally less active in cold weather. Eating root vegetables in soups or roasted provides healthy carbs as well as the comfort of hot foods. Eating citrus in winter helps prevent colds with an extra helping of vitamin C.

Reap the Benefits

Local seasonal foods are an important part of a healthy diet for all the reasons listed above because they:

1. provide what we need when we need it, another powerful example of how our bodies and our natural environment work in sync to keep us healthy.
2. assist us in eating a varied diet, which is important to ensure we get all the nutrients we need in a variety of combinations.
3. are a double bargain, providing the biggest bang for our buck in nutrition, freshness, and taste, while our wallet gets a big win with a lower price.
4. support local farmers, local jobs and communities.
5. are not transported from hundreds or thousands of miles away, which greatly diminishes the impact on the environment.

GETTING REACQUAINTED WITH YOUR KITCHEN

Any taste, texture, or favorite food recipe can be recreated in many different ways. The key to feeding your body for health is to start with whole, unprocessed foods as the main ingredients—locally grown for freshness, taste, and low environmental impact, and organic when available and affordable. Then go where your heart and your taste buds take you! As long as you eat a wide variety of plant-based whole foods and are mindful to reduce the amount of salt, sugar, and oil you may add in preparing them, enjoy to your heart's content.

Although I have always loved to eat, and to enjoy what I eat, I always struggled with cooking! Cooking for me was work I didn't enjoy, and it is hard to do something well if you don't enjoy it. One of the reasons I didn't like cooking was my lack of confidence in the kitchen. I tried to follow recipes but invariably in the process I'd overlook a step entirely, do something in the wrong order, or discover in the midst of the process that I was missing an ingredient. My results were an occasional hit and a lot of miss.

Learning the difference between feeding myself and eating, along with the desire to enjoy the best state of health I can create for myself and my family, led me to start experimenting again with cooking. The other reason is that although healthy and delicious plant-based restaurants are becoming more popular, they are not yet mainstream. Although you may be surprised to find some very good ones in your area, they are not common outside of metropolitan areas where the market is growing fast enough to sustain them. Those of us who live in places like New York, Chicago, Atlanta, and Los Angeles are blessed with many amazing options. My hometown Houston market is small and growing, and although limited in number, offers some very good vegan eateries. Even though they are generally priced fairly based on the quality of the ingredients and the care they take when preparing the food, you can certainly make great plant-based food at home for less.

For all these reasons, I had to overcome my insecurity about cooking and start to hang out in my own kitchen! And guess what? I discovered that, just as I had previously approached eating in an unconscious way, I had been approaching food preparation in the same manner. I saw it as a chore that I wanted to finish in as short a time as possible. I did not take the time to make sure I had every-thing I needed, and then I tried to rush through the process, which led to missteps. And because eating something I would enjoy was my main focus, not feeding my health, I could do that quicker and easier by getting take-out.

Now feeding myself means providing delicious, healthy foods for my body so that it feels good, functions well, avoids disease, and ages slowly. Feeding myself is a mindful process that includes the soul satisfaction of experiencing food with all the senses—sight, smell, taste, texture, and even sound, as in the crunch of a crisp, juicy apple in the fall. All are important to enjoying the foods I eat. In order to eat fresh, whole foods on a budget, and especially if you want organic, you will spend most of your supermarket shopping time in the fresh produce section and prepare your food at home.

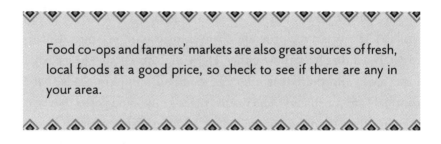

Food co-ops and farmers' markets are also great sources of fresh, local foods at a good price, so check to see if there are any in your area.

For all these reasons, we have to get reacquainted with our kitchen as the place where good health meets good taste. Those who are comfortable in the kitchen will find adapting to vegan recipes or making healthier choices in preparing familiar foods surprisingly easy. Those like myself who largely avoided cooking will want to start with simpler recipes that are quick, easy, and tasty. Some of the best need only a few ingredients. Take the time to make a list before going grocery shopping so you won't forget anything. I've learned to assemble everything I need and lay it all out on my kitchen counter—tools, bowls, colander, whatever—before I start preparing a dish. Then I prep the vegetables or fruit and line up all the ingredients. I had to learn to go about the whole process consciously. And guess what? The results get better and better, simply because I am focused on what I am doing, and I am motivated. I was someone who never thought I would be confident in the kitchen, so if I can do it, you certainly can too!

In a few months, I put away my favorite recipes and, for the most part, I could make good food without them. And then it happened! One day one of the ingredients for a raw organic vegan pesto sauce which I love—fresh basil, fresh garlic, nutritional yeast, raw pine nuts, lemon juice and vegetable broth—was missing. I forgot that I had used the last of the raw pine nuts the last time I made it. I was irritated at first for forgetting I was out, and also at the thought of stopping in the middle of getting dinner ready, to go to the store to find it. Then I pulled out my tablet and googled raw vegan pesto. Voila! There was a recipe using walnuts instead of pine nuts. Unfortunately, I didn't have those either. I looked in my cabinet to see what I did have, and there was a bag of sprouted pumpkin seeds that I routinely ate for snacks. The result was a really good pesto that was even healthier than the original recipe because of the nutritional content of the pumpkin seeds. The whole experience was so gratifying!

From that point on, I started to be more spontaneous and challenge myself to create meals from whatever I had on hand. This was actually fun. My confidence increased along with my enjoyment of my time in the kitchen, and for the first time in my life, I started to like the food I made better than what I could buy. Be bold and creative in your kitchen. Start with a basic recipe like the ones you will find in the back of this book, and then improvise to suit your family's preferences.

Many friends tell stories about making a meal that everyone enjoys, and at the end seeing the surprise on the faces of friends or family when they tell them it was all plant-based.

RAW FOOD ADVANTAGE

Raw vegetables and fruits are indispensable for achieving your best health. I shared in chapter 3 that several years ago my cardiologist recommended a 100 percent raw, plant-based diet as a nutritional cure for my hypertension and cardiovascular disease. Although I initially thought, *No way*, the prospect of staying on drugs for the rest of my life made me reconsider. And now, even though my blood pressure is normal, and my other heart disease symptoms are either reversed or improved, raw foods still make up 70 to 80 percent of what I eat daily. Remember that what we enjoy is a product of what we are accustomed to, what we grew up with, and what we are surrounded by. I eat mostly raw fruits and vegetables now because I appreciate and prefer them. I have become accustomed to their variety of flavors, textures, fragrances, and vibrant colors that are a beautiful feast for the eyes and the spirit. I have expanded, not narrowed, my preparation options, because I used to think that food like corn, collards, and zucchini *had* to be cooked.

The benefits of eating raw or live foods are:

1. Enzymes in raw foods are necessary for the body to absorb and utilize food nutrients. These same enzymes are destroyed by cooking, which explains the growing probiotic supplement market resulting from the lack of fresh whole food in our diet.
2. Because fresh raw whole foods are more flavorful, you need less salt, sugar, and oil to enhance their taste. And the higher the raw food content in your diet, the less room there is for processed foods.
3. Raw vegetables, fruit, nuts, and seeds are healing because of the integrity of their nutritional value and also because of what they do not contain (added salt, sugar, oil, fillers, and chemicals)

4. Raw fresh foods are beautiful with every vivid color of the rainbow. The colors in food are indicators of their nutritional content and add to their enjoyment.

Salads

Fresh salads made from an infinite variety of vegetables, fruit, nuts, seeds, grains, and seasonings are a very easy, quick, and convenient way to keep the raw food content in your diet high. Keep lots of green leafy vegetables like kale, spinach, baby lettuces, romaine, arugula, radicchio, collards, red and green cabbage, bok choy, and many others in your fridge. Add fruit, tomatoes, avocados, red onion, celery, sweet peppers, carrots, zucchini, squash, or any vegetable your heart desires. For an extra punch of protein, add almonds, walnuts, cashews, pistachios, pecans, or cooked rice, quinoa, farro, garbanzo beans, or black-eyed peas. To ramp up the nutrition with omega-3 and omega-6, sprinkle on raw pumpkin, sesame, or chia seeds. For even more flavor, add raisins, dried cranberries, or other dried fruit to the mix.

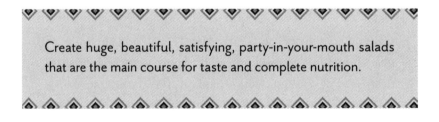

Create huge, beautiful, satisfying, party-in-your-mouth salads that are the main course for taste and complete nutrition.

Please try a couple of my favorites in the recipe section along with some awesome raw treats like raw vegan pesto, great as a dip or pasta sauce!

Smoothies

God bless whoever invented the fruit smoothie! They are virtually impossible to screw up and taste amazing, no matter what combination of fruits you throw in. And, unlike juicing, you get all the fiber, which makes them filling and satisfying. The fiber also helps avoid a sugar spike compared to fruit juices, which are stripped of the pulp and fiber. I make them by the pitcher and try to keep this treat on hand much of the time. A quick stir and they're as good as when they came out of the blender.

You really don't need a recipe for smoothies. Some of my all-time favorites are mango, pineapple, and peach with fresh-squeezed orange juice; and watermelon, strawberry, and grape, also with a splash of fresh-squeezed orange juice. I also like adding a vegetable or two to my fruit smoothies. Kale, spinach, carrots, and beets are some of my favorites. I tried making all-vegetable smoothies, which for me were a bust. The flavor was good, but I prefer to eat my veggies, or to add greens, beets or carrots to fruit smoothies. Check out my delicious pineapple green smoothie in the recipe section, my favorite go-to drink for an immune system boost!

Sautés

For someone like me who never liked to cook, one of the most exciting discoveries was the quick vegetable sauté. They are about as versatile in their combinations as a smoothie and are very quick, delicious, and satisfying over brown rice, polenta, quinoa, farro, or other grains. I like to vary the flavor with spice combinations to achieve a Creole, Asian, Mexican, or Italian taste experience. The key is to start with a base to create a flavorful sauce. My favorite is a combination of onion with chopped tomatoes, celery, garlic, parsley or cilantro. Early on I used vegan bouillon cubes (Not Chicken and Not Beef were my favorites), but do check labels to make sure there is no MSG, known to trigger headache, heart palpitations, flushing, sweating, asthma, or numbness in some people. As my confidence in the kitchen grew, I found that I could create the same tastes with fresh herbs and whatever spice combination I'm in the mood for.

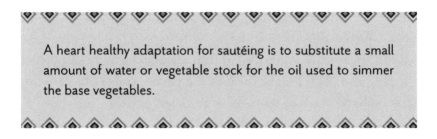

A heart healthy adaptation for sautéing is to substitute a small amount of water or vegetable stock for the oil used to simmer the base vegetables.

If you use oil, choose a high heat-tolerant one like almond or grape-seed. I make my base by simmering onion and tomatoes with spices and a little water, just long enough for the flavors to blend and the sauce to thicken slightly, or about five minutes. Then I throw in zucchini, carrots, celery, corn spinach, chard, or whatever I have in the fridge with my spices, for five to ten minutes longer, and voila! I put the carrots in first and the spinach or chard last because of the different cooking times. I start my brown rice in the rice cooker beforehand, and because it lasts for four to six days in the fridge, I make enough for two or three meals. Or I make quinoa or polenta, which take twelve to fifteen minutes. If you are heart healthy enough and like the taste, you can drizzle a little cold-pressed extra virgin olive oil over the sauté immediately after cooking and let it rest, with the remaining heat helping to absorb the flavor of the oil. One of my favorites, sautéed collards with cherry tomatoes, onion, and peppers, is found in the recipe section.

Soups

Oh, my God, how I love soups! I particularly enjoy hearty soups with beans, lentils, or peas. Soups are another great-tasting food that is nearly foolproof. For those not-there-yet wannabe gourmet cooks like myself, it's helpful to start with a basic recipe, and then you can improvise. Soups are also quick and hassle free because you don't want to overcook the vegetables.

One of my favorites is a vegetarian gumbo that is a cross between a Louisiana gumbo and a West African *soupe kandia*, which is very similar to its Louisiana cousin but made with red palm oil. Red palm oil, like coconut oil, contains saturated fat. I prefer to use almond or grape-seed oil which are both high heat-tolerant, or to leave the oil out altogether. With gumbos, the base, which is called a roux, is the key.

The trick to making a good roux without sautéing in oil is to heat the flour (I like garbanzo flour for high protein and taste) and roux spice mix in a dry skillet to brown them, and then add water or vegetable stock to finish a nice dark brown roux. Or make in the traditional way starting with a high heat-tolerant oil like almond, along with your flour and roux seasoning. Next, add onion, garlic, and spices and simmer until the base thickens. Then add whatever vegetables and seasonings you like, as you would with any gumbo. I've included my Senegalese gumbo recipe, vegan style, in the recipe section. Remember that soups, like salads, are a perfect opportunity for creative expression. Don't be afraid to add ingredients you love.

Steaming

Steaming vegetables is a really good way to enjoy minimally cooked foods for a quick hot meal while retaining many of the nutrients, color, and flavor otherwise lost when they are boiled or exposed to high heat for an extended period of time. Brussels sprouts, carrots, bok choy, rutabaga, turnips, cabbage, beets, potatoes, and leafy greens are great steamed. Use a pot with a steamer basket that fits on top and is covered with a lid to keep in the steam. The pot is filled with about an inch of water and brought to a slow boil. Then place the vegetables in the steamer basket and sprinkle on the spices and herbs to add flavor and interest.

I sometimes spray a tiny amount of liquid aminos like Bragg's over the vegetables, or marinate them the night before to further enhance the flavor. They are also really good just naked, and most take only five minutes or so to achieve a tender result with the colors—an indication of the food's vitality—still vibrant.

If you don't have a steamer, just fill a pot with an inch of water, put three golf-ball-sized wads of aluminum foil in a triangle on the bottom, and place a heat-safe plate on top of the aluminum balls so that it doesn't touch the water. Once the water boils, place your veggies on the plate, sprinkle seasoning if you like, and then cover the pot with a lid.

One health benefit of steaming is that more water-soluble vitamins like C and B are retained because they do not come in direct contact with the boiling water. These vitamins are important to keeping our immune systems strong, and B vitamins promote healthy brain function and help the body process glucose (sugar). Light steaming requires no oil, which means you do not add fat and calories to the food. Light steaming for short periods of time preserves healthy food properties better than other cooking methods and better protects food enzymes. It is a healthy, quick, easy, delicious, and colorful way to add variety to your meal.

Baking

Because baking is done at temperatures above 120 degrees Fahrenheit, and usually for more than twenty minutes, it does not protect the nutrients and enzymes so abundant in raw whole foods. One interesting alternative is to use a dehydrator to achieve flavor and taste similar to baking, but with temperatures under 120 degrees. Dehydrating foods will still not protect vitamin C and B vitamins, which are sensitive to heat as well as water. It does, however, preserve more nutrients than baking at high heat. You can dehydrate fruits like apples, berries, bananas, peaches, and mangoes. Once dehydrated, they will have a chewy texture and a flavor concentrated from the loss of water content. They can be eaten as snacks or used as a tasty addition to salads and other dishes. Vegetables like tomatoes, mushrooms, onions, greens, and carrots can also be dehydrated. They will be crispy and can be eaten as snacks or added to other dishes. Good home size dehydrators are available online for $200–300.

Enjoying baked foods, like breads and desserts, is something most of us can occasionally do as part of a healthy diet, as long as we pay attention to the ingredients and use healthier sweeteners, fats, whole grain flours, and other ingredients. I've included one of my favorite really simple fruit crisp recipes in the recipe section. And if you're up for a little challenge, I've added the recipe for my gluten-free, whole grain, seeded bread packed with heart-healthy ingredients. I never thought I would take the time to bake my own bread, but once you taste it, you'll see that it's well worth the effort!

HOW TO EAT OUT
Gaming a Restaurant Menu

Because most of us eat out from time to time, and usually not at vegan restaurants, another absolutely critical skill I learned along the way is how to "game" a mainstream restaurant menu. This is a kind of modern day foraging which I now enjoy as a challenge. Here's how it works:

1. Scan the menu for ingredients, particularly those that are listed in the salad and "sides" section of the menu. These are the necessary and generally underappreciated components of a typical menu where the vegetables and fruits are found. This does not work at a fast food restaurant where everything is precooked and prepackaged and there is likely

nothing unprocessed, not GMO, not to mention organic in the place to begin with. But that is not where we, as mindful eaters, will spend our time or our money.

2. Pick an item, usually a salad, from the menu that has the most ingredients you like. When the server asks for your order, say you will have the "garden" or "whatever it's called" salad without the ingredients you don't want (cheese, bacon, egg) and substitute other things you've found on the menu (nuts, avocado slices, sesame or pumpkin seeds, beets, red onion, artichokes). Ask for vinegar and oil, if you choose, rather than prepared dressings because typically nobody but the chef knows what's in them, and many use raw egg as a thickener. Let them know to upsize if necessary because this is your main course.

3. Then for your "sides" pick whatever you like: a baked potato, roasted potatoes, or any vegetable you see on the menu that is not prepared with dairy, animal fat or broth, or fried. Roasted vegetables are usually a safe choice but ensure that they're made with olive oil, not butter. Steamed veggies are usually another safe choice. French fries are also vegan, but we won't go there!

4. Listen carefully now: you don't have to skip dessert! Scour the menu again for berries or other fruit that may be a side or a garnish. My favorite is to get a dish of strawberries, blueberries, raspberries, or plain nuts and drizzle with a little honey, which they almost always have. Or I get a cup of herbal tea with lemon and honey for a bit of sweetness to finish the meal, and I have my dessert later when I get home.

This works in almost any restaurant with a real kitchen, as most offer some fresh—and sometimes even organic—choices. And even if you can't have organic, you will have a fresh, colorful, interesting, enjoyable, well-prepared meal.

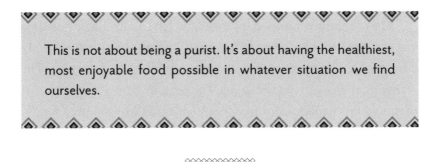

This is not about being a purist. It's about having the healthiest, most enjoyable food possible in whatever situation we find ourselves.

◇◇◇◇◇◇◇◇◇◇◇◇

I've even had a couple of restaurants comment that they might want to include my "creation" on the menu. Not bad for someone who never thought I had any talent in the kitchen! And even if they don't put it on the menu, they begin to get the message that there is a growing demand and market for fresh real food.

Beautiful Dinner on the Road

Speaking of repurposing restaurant menu items, one of my earliest and best memories of my journey to a plant-based diet happened in, of all places, Tulsa, Oklahoma. Picture this: I've spent the whole day at a business conference and trade show. Because of a mix-up in the reservation, my hotel is not downtown near the Convention Center, but a remote location with the same hotel chain thirty miles outside of Tulsa in a suburban area I had never heard of. After getting lost and nearly giving up, I finally find the place, check in, and find myself frustrated and hungry. I get to the restaurant about eight thirty, and there's only one other guest in the whole place—not a good sign. The waiter seats me and provides the menu, which includes some Italian items. When he comes to take my order, I explain that I am vegetarian (at the time) and that I'd found a couple of items on the menu that I would like to modify. I then ordered the citrus salad with mixed baby greens and almonds. For the main course I selected an entrée with chicken and polenta, however I did not want the chicken. I asked if they could instead sauté vegetables to serve over the polenta.

The other diner finished his meal and left. As I waited, I became less concerned with dinner and wished instead that I were already done with the day and heading to my room like the other guest. The waiter then brought out the salad. The presentation was nice, but at that point my expectations were not high, and I was too tired for the food to be my main concern. I thanked him then took a bite. Hmm . . . nice, crisp greens, light lemony dressing, layered with subtle hints of herbs and seasonings, some of which I could not immediately identify. Suddenly I was hungry again, and this salad was exquisite!

Just as I finished the salad, the waiter appeared with my improvised main course. Again, I immediately noticed a very nice presentation. The medley of brightly colored vegetables—red and yellow peppers, zucchini ribbons, sliced fresh mushrooms, onion, fresh garlic and tomato—was nestled atop the polenta and drizzled in a sauce which appeared to have been created in the process of sautéing the vegetables in olive oil. I took a bite and, *mama mia*, all my attention shifted to that dish. The polenta was flavorful and the perfect consistency. The outside was slightly seared to a delicate dark golden color, the center firm but moist. Here in the middle of God knows where was a blessing in the form of a wonderful meal. I called over the waiter to order a glass of sauvignon blanc and completely forgot how tired I had been. I gave thanks that wines are vegan!

I ate slowly and deliberately, savoring every forkful. I took the last bite with a touch of regret. When the waiter appeared again to ask if I enjoyed the meal, he smiled because he already knew the answer. I told him that it was absolutely delightful, and as he cleared the table, I asked him to give my compliments to the chef. A few moments later a very young man in chef's attire came over to my table. He thanked me for the kind words, and I told him how much I enjoyed the dinner and that I really appreciated his flexibility in creating it for me. He said he had just graduated from Oklahoma University in their culinary arts program. He went on to say that he took a special course in vegetarian and vegan cooking and that this had been an opportunity for him to draw on that experience. We chatted for a few moments, and then I left for my room, having experienced what was quite possibly the highlight of my day. And to think I almost stopped at Subway for an iceberg lettuce salad a block before reaching that hotel!

Vegan in a Steakhouse

Here's my favorite menu-gaming example, which happened in a popular Houston steakhouse chain, of all places. I was there for a business lunch and figured I'd pick a salad for my meal. But every salad, side dish, and other menu item came with beef, chicken, pork, or shrimp either in it or on it. I happened to be hungrier than I realized and didn't want to leave the same way. I looked the menu up and down, scanning for whatever I could find to make a really good and satisfying salad. The first thing I always rule out is iceberg lettuce. It is one of the least nutritious vegetables, is mass produced, and is the most common "green" in most commercial kitchens because it is cheap.

So that day on the Saltgrass Steakhouse menu I saw a fresh spinach salad that came with a choice of steak or chicken strips. The fresh spinach, although certainly not organic, was encouraging. Then I saw an entrée with avocado slices, another salad with red onion and pecans. And then I hit pay dirt. There was an appetizer of pico de gallo, a staple usually offered at area Mexican food eateries. It is a mixture of fresh onion, jalapeño, tomato, and cilantro, in this case served in true Southwest style with fried corn chips. When the waiter approached to take our orders, I asked my companion to go first. This is an important part of the process, since what I improvise will take a minute, not because it is difficult, but because the waiter will have to shift gears, and some are better at it than others. When it was my turn I asked if I could have a modified entrée size spinach salad. I then asked for the salad without the cheese, croutons, steak, or chicken, and asked instead to add avocado and pecans for extra protein, red onions, and the magical spicy pico de gallo, which I love on just about anything. I also asked for balsamic vinegar instead of the prepared dressings, along with some fresh lemon to enhance the flavor.

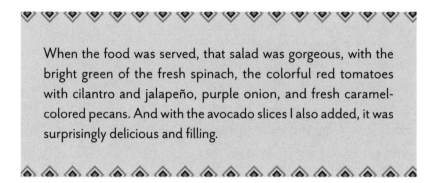

When the food was served, that salad was gorgeous, with the bright green of the fresh spinach, the colorful red tomatoes with cilantro and jalapeño, purple onion, and fresh caramel-colored pecans. And with the avocado slices I also added, it was surprisingly delicious and filling.

I had a satisfying lunch, good conversation, and left feeling really positive about the entire experience. I enjoyed it so much that I started to look forward to the next restaurant challenge!

The moral of the story is that when we are mindful, we can discover abundance in almost any situation. Even though the standard American diet is poor overall from a nutritional standpoint, in the US, most of us have more choice in how and what we feed ourselves than the majority of people around the world. The best and most uplifting food experiences often happen when least expected and in the most unlikely places. It's just a matter of staying present in the moment and aware of the choices all around us.

Living and feeding ourselves consciously is grounded in respect for our own bodies, for our fellow Earth inhabitants, both human and animal, and for the natural environment on which we all depend. We understand that a healthy body depends on a healthy planet. The important thing to remember is that every positive change we make in what and how we feed ourselves, no matter how small, has a cumulative positive impact on restoring our environment as well as our own good health, and that we don't have to choose between great health and great food.

CHAPTER 7

Making Healthy Choices

"What most people don't realize is that food is more than calories, it's information. It actually contains messages that connect to every cell in the body."

—Dr. Mark Hyman, physician and author

OPENING OUR MINDS TO THE unlimited possibilities to feed our bodies in amazingly delicious and healthy ways helps us begin to see this same abundance in other areas of our lives. It feeds our creativity and our confidence that everything we need to achieve our dreams is available to us, including good health. Further, it suggests that this is best accomplished by respecting our natural environment, by protecting and living in concert with it.

All of the healthy choices offered here have been included in healthy diets for thousands of years in various parts of the world. They are plant based and minimally processed or unprocessed to retain their nutrition, disease-fighting properties, and peak flavors. Many of these foods have become new favorites, especially when combined with seasonal fresh produce in an endless variety of ways.

SUGAR AND ALTERNATIVE SWEETENERS

There is probably more confusion about sugars and sweeteners than any other component of our diet, and for good reason. As we discussed earlier, our bodies from very early in our evolution were programmed to love sweet foods. Let's start with the basics. The most widely used sweetener, refined cane sugar, was not widely available until the eighteenth century. It is made from sugar cane, but with modern manufacturing methods, it is highly processed and stripped of any nutrients.

Dr. Robert Lustig, co-author in 2009 of the American Heart Association's guideline on sugar intake, presented a paper that same year entitled "Sugar: The Bitter Truth." It was posted on YouTube and has been viewed over six million times, quite impressive for a ninety-minute scientific lecture intended for medical students. In the video, he refers to refined sugar as a toxin, a poison. It is not a poison with an immediate toxic effect, but rather one that manifests over time. This lecture, and books by Lustig and others, maintain refined sugar is not only devoid of any nutritional value, but that it actually leaches nutrients from the body.

Continuing medical research on metabolic syndrome, the group of factors that are predictive markers for the development of obesity, heart disease, diabetes, and cancer, points to inflammation and insulin resistance caused by eating habits common in the SAD diet.

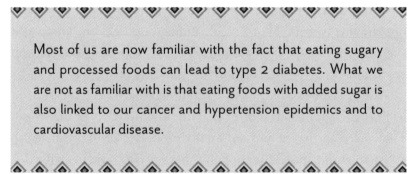

Most of us are now familiar with the fact that eating sugary and processed foods can lead to type 2 diabetes. What we are not as familiar with is that eating foods with added sugar is also linked to our cancer and hypertension epidemics and to cardiovascular disease.

This includes white table sugar as well as brown or raw sugar and processed cane, beet, and coconut sugars. High-fructose corn syrup is added to so many processed foods that it has specifically been linked to the growth of many diseases including heart disease, diabetes, obesity, and cancers. It can be difficult to recognize from reading food labels when a product contains added sugar because they are not always clear. You have to look for things like dextrose, glucose, lactose, maltose, and sucrose to be sure.

Sugars with a high glycemic index, meaning they are quickly absorbed into the blood stream, are particularly troublesome. Without a doubt, eliminating or limiting added sugar is a change you can make to protect and enhance your health. The practical advice from the medical experts is that the healthiest sugars are those that are eaten as part of whole fruits or vegetables because the fiber in the whole food buffers the rate at which the fructose or sugar is absorbed in the bloodstream.

For instance, if you drink orange juice, there is a sugar spike in your bloodstream, whereas if you eat the whole orange, this does not happen because of the fiber. See the table below for the definition of low, medium, and high ratings.

GLYCEMIC INDEX RATINGS
Low Glycemic Index: 0–55
Medium Glycemic Index: 56–69
High Glycemic Index: 70–100

We are not likely to eliminate sweeteners, nor do we have to as long as we limit our use and intake. When choosing a sweetener, you will ideally want one whose nutrients are intact, and whose glycemic index is low, meaning it will absorb more slowly into the blood stream. It is also important to note the fructose content, because this form of sugar, found naturally in fruit, can be detrimental when separated from the fruit flesh and consumed in large quantities, as in fruit juices. It is also the type of sugar found in agave. Fructose is processed only by the liver and can contribute to insulin resistance. And how about the artificial sugar substitutes advertised and available in every grocery store and restaurant? You don't want to go there. These products are typically not foods, but food-like substances created in a chemistry lab. Please see the chart below for a comparison summary of the glycemic index and nutrient profile of popular cane sugar alternatives.[22]

Plant-Based Sweetner Comparison

SWEETENER	TYPE OF SUGAR	GLYCEMIC INDEX	CARBOHYDRATES PER 20 GRAMS	NUTRITIVE CALORIC
Natural Stevia	Natural	0	0	No
Monk Fruit	Natural	0	20	No
Maple Syrup	Natural	54	13	Yes
Coconut Sugar	Natural	35	20	Yes
Raw Honey	Raw	58	16	Yes
Raw Agave	Raw	19	15	Yes
Brown Rice Syrup	Natural	98	15	Yes
Xylitol	Sugar Alcohol	7	20	Yes

Honey

Many people use honey as a natural sugar substitute. Its advantages are that in its organic, raw, and unrefined state, it has significant antibacterial properties. It counters seasonal allergies by exposing us to small amounts of pollen, which help desensitize us to the greater amounts in the air we breathe, similar to how vaccinations work. Research published by the National Institute of Health (NIH) reports that raw honey is effective in treating simple burns or infections by applying it directly to the injury to form a barrier. In this way it blocks out air and aids healing with its antimicrobial effect. It is said to reduce healing time, redness, and swelling similar to antibiotics.

On the downside, although many people like the taste and health benefits of honey, its distinctive taste may alter the flavor of foods when added. It also has a glycemic index only slightly less than refined sugar, which means it can cause blood sugar spikes. In addition, it is not very suitable for cooking and baking. Raw honey should be used with caution by anyone who has a compromised immune system and should never be given to babies less than one year old due to the risk of infant botulism from bacterial spores.

Stevia

Another popular sweetener is stevia, which comes from the leaves of the plant of the same name. It is native to Paraguay and has been used there as a sweetener for beverages and medicines since the sixteenth century. Available in liquid or powder form, stevia can be a good choice for diabetics, or for anyone concerned about regulating blood glucose levels. It has been shown not to cause blood sugar or insulin elevation and is considered a "zero calorie" food because it is poorly absorbed by the digestive tract and is excreted in the urine. It has an intense sweetness, but it also has a noticeable aftertaste that some people do not like. I find the liquid form very suitable as a sweetness enhancer for fruit smoothies or other naturally sweet foods without adding calories. When I use it in this way, the aftertaste is not noticeable.

Based on the source and purity of stevia in the marketplace, and how it is compounded, stevia could also help in lowering blood pressure and regulating heart rate when taken in higher doses. You should contact your health care professional before using stevia in this manner. It also contains several antioxidants including kaempferol, which can reduce the risk of pancreatic cancer by as much as 23 percent. Stevia is safe for the general population, including children.

Raw Coconut Sugar

This sweetener has a mild taste, which I find similar to brown cane sugar. It is unbleached, unrefined, and gluten free. Because the sap is evaporated at low temperatures in processing, the enzymes and nutrients are not destroyed, which technically makes it a raw food. The sap has a very low glycemic index (GI 35) and is an abundant source of minerals, seventeen amino acids, vitamin C, and B vitamins, as well as having a nearly neutral pH. Sucrose is the major component of coconut sap and also coconut crystals at 70–79 percent. It also has about 3–5 percent glucose and 3–5 percent fructose, depending on the age and variety of the trees from which it is harvested. The fructose content is lower than sugar, which is a positive because fructose can only be metabolized by the liver and can contribute to insulin resistance.

Coconut crystals are also made from the sap of the coconut tree flower, but the sap is boiled to evaporate it, which destroys the enzymes. Otherwise, the composition and health benefits are similar. Coconut crystals or raw nectar can be used like table sugar in teas, cereals, cooking, or baking. It is typically sustainably harvested, which makes its appeal even sweeter.

Raw Agave

Agave in its raw form is a live food harvested from the agave plant, which grows in the deserts of Mexico. Until recently the agave plant was much better known as the main ingredient in the production of tequila. Its sweetness is three times that of refined sugar with no aftertaste. It is also relatively inexpensive and can be used in baking and cooking.

It contains trace amounts of fructans, commonly found in foods like asparagus, artichokes, and green beans. Some research has shown that fructans may reduce fat and cholesterol absorption in the intestine, but there is likely not enough in agave alone to cause that effect.

The downside of agave is its high fructose content, which can vary widely from brand to brand, based on the method of processing. This attribute has led many people to seek other options because agave may promote insulin resistance.

Maple Syrup

Native Americans processed the sap from maple trees into syrup long before the arrival of European settlers. Used in moderation, as with any sweetener, maple syrup can be beneficial by helping to lower inflammation and supplying some trace minerals and nutrients. And it has a distinctive flavor enjoyed by most people. Cane sugar and maple syrup are both about 65 percent sucrose, but maple syrup has a glycemic index score of 54, slightly better than table sugar at 65.

Another factor that makes these two sweeteners very different is how they are made and the environmental impact. Maple syrup is produced by boiling the tree sap, heating it to a temperature of just over two hundred degrees, and then filtering the resulting syrup to remove any impurities, which is a fairly simple process. Although some describe it as raw, that is only by comparison to cane sugar, which goes through an extensive process of washing, milling, juice extraction, filtration, purification, and condensation in order to produce sugar crystals. This extreme processing eliminates any nutritional content in cane sugar.

Molasses

Molasses is made by extracting the juice from sugar cane and then boiling to concentrate it. This first produces a syrup known in the South as cane syrup, which I remember eating on pancakes as a kid. There is a second, and then a third boiling which produces the dark blackstrap molasses which has a strong distinctive flavor.

Unlike highly refined sugars, it contains significant amounts of vitamin B-6 and minerals, including calcium, magnesium, iron, and manganese; one tablespoon provides up to 20 percent of the recommended daily value of each of those nutrients. Blackstrap is also a good source of potassium and has long been sold as a dietary supplement. However, remember that molasses is a form of refined sugar. It has nutrients and minerals but also a high glycemic index. In addition, it contains 20 percent or so of fructose and another 20 percent sucrose. Because of these factors it must be used very sparingly, like honey, cane sugar, agave, or any sweetener removed from its natural source.

Moderation Is Key

When it comes to sweeteners, there is much confusing information, conflicting information, one-sided information, and plain old exaggeration of beneficial aspects of a product while ignoring detrimental ones. I have to say this was a learning experience that required checking multiple sources, those touting a particular type of sweetener and those panning it. As a result, some of my earlier assumptions I no longer hold as true. In particular, a few years ago, I embraced agave as a raw food; however, the high fructose content is not desirable due to potential impact on the liver.

My goal of sharing facts with you that are useful and relevant to making good health decisions is anything but clear cut when it comes to sweeteners. The simple truth that did emerge from all of the articles, studies, research and blogs is this: *Our mothers got it right. Don't eat too much sugar.* The key takeaway is that any sweetener added to food, even natural ones, must be used in moderation. The only exception is eating sugar as it naturally occurs in whole fruits and vegetables. The failsafe there is that it's difficult to eat enough volume of whole foods for the sugar they contain to harm us. Remember how long it takes to chew a stalk of sugar cane!

Used in moderation, organic, raw, or minimally processed sweeteners can support our overall health, wellness, and enjoyment of the foods we eat. There are many choices that will delight us with their versatility as table sweeteners, and in cooking and baking, that are healthier than white table sugar. They are a perfect example of how a mindful approach to food can provide great taste, variety, and the nutrition our bodies need. The notion that you must sacrifice one for the other is a myth. *For those who are diagnosed as diabetic or prediabetic, please consult your health care provider before adding any form of sweetener to your diet.*

PLENTIFUL PROTEIN

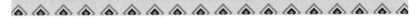

One of the greatest misconceptions about vegetarian and vegan lifestyles is that it is difficult to provide the body with sufficient protein.

Some of us may remember the Seven Basic Food Group posters in junior high and being taught that we needed to choose from each group daily for good health. Although clearly misguided in light of the nutritional knowledge available to us today, the popular concept of a healthy diet is still rooted in the teachings of fifty years ago. The belief that we can only get protein from animal sources is still strong. First of all, every plant has protein. That's right, every plant.

A paper examining the quality and utility of animal and plant protein sources entitled "Which is Best?" was presented at an International Society of Sports Nutrition Symposium in 2004 and published by the National Center for Biotechnology Information (NCBI). The article states, "For proteins to be used by the body, they need to be metabolized into their simplest form, amino acids. There have been twenty amino acids identified that are needed for human growth and metabolism. Twelve of these amino acids (eleven in children) are termed nonessential, meaning that they can be synthesized by our body and do not need to be consumed in the diet. The remaining amino acids cannot be synthesized in the body and are described as essential, meaning that they need to be consumed in our diets."

It goes on to say, "Typically, all dietary animal protein sources are considered to be complete proteins. That is, a protein that contains all of the essential amino acids. Proteins from vegetable sources are incomplete in that they are generally lacking one or two essential amino acids. Thus, someone who desires to get their protein from vegetable sources (i.e. vegetarian) will need to consume a variety of vegetables, fruits, grains, and legumes to ensure consumption of all essential amino acids. As such, individuals are able to achieve necessary protein requirements without consuming beef, poultry, or dairy."[23]

In other words, when we eat an animal, the animal has already eaten plant nutrition and converted it into protein containing all nine essential amino acids, which are used by its muscles and organs for growth. We eat the flesh of the animal and the complete protein with all nine essential amino acids it contains. Since an individual plant does not contain all nine essential amino acids, by eating a variety of them, each high in some and low in others, our bodies achieve the same result of complete protein. And isn't this how we eat naturally by combining foods? The myth that it is difficult to get enough protein through plant sources is not based on the reality of how humans eat and overlooks the intelligent, symbiotic, and complex interactions our bodies have with our food.

Multiple studies over the last several decades have shown that protein from plant sources can be complete and sufficient to meet the body's needs. Many plant-based foods like grains, nuts, legumes, and many vegetables have significant protein content. Eating legumes like beans and peas in combination with whole grains like brown rice, quinoa, or corn creates a complete protein source.

Fish, relatively speaking, is a healthier choice than red meat, pork, or chicken, in that it contains fewer harmful fats, and some varieties of

> The most important way plant-based protein provides a significant advantage over animal protein is that it does not contain the harmful fats, cholesterol, and triglycerides found in meats.

oily fish like salmon are a source of healthy omega-3 fatty acids which promote heart function. Omega-3 fatty acids also support the brain and eyes, which are made up of the long-chain fatty acids DHA and EPA that omega-3 produces. One thing that all animal foods, including fish, have in common, however, is the inflammatory response they trigger in the human body. This becomes more of a problem as we age and our immune systems are less robust. At that point, inflammation can contribute to an accelerated aging process. Conditions like heart disease, arthritis, cancer, and autoimmune disorders can be triggered by this inflammatory reaction to animal protein.

As someone who has eaten a vegetarian diet for most of my adult life, and who is interested in nutrition, I wanted to know how eating only plants might show up in my own diagnostic blood tests which are used to check for imbalances, deficiencies, and healthy or harmful levels of certain blood characteristics. It is generally a kind of report card on underlying health factors that compares individual results to a statistical norm. For each of these comprehensive blood panels I have had for the past several years, my protein level is consistently in the normal range—and that is based on data for the population as a whole, which includes significantly more meat eaters than vegans or vegetarians. I am at the same place most meat eaters are with respect to the amount of protein I get.

What most vegans are challenged with is maintaining a healthy level of B-12. Bacteria containing Vitamin B-12 are found in the clumps of dirt around grass roots, and in traces of feces eaten accidently by cows and other animals as they eat grasses and other plants, so long as the soil is not deficient in the mineral cobalt.

Chickens eat the same bacteria when pecking in the dirt for worms and other insects. When meat eaters consume them they also get the benefit of the B-12 in their systems. However, because much of our soil has been depleted of cobalt, and because most food animals now come from factory farms where they may never be exposed to dirt, let alone a natural diet, 95 percent of the B-12 supplements manufactured are given to farm animals. Most meat eaters today also benefit from B-12 supplements, secondhand. Our ancestors got plenty of B-12 from the rich soils that had not been over-farmed and by drinking water from streams or rivers that contained B-12-producing bacteria, with or without meat in their diet. Vegans and those eating a primarily plant-based diet today do well to take B-12 supplements to ensure optimal long-term health.

Soy

There have been many articles written about societies where people who live to be a hundred years of age are common, and overall life expectancy exceeds the norm in the US. These societies have primarily plant-based dietary traditions in which meat is not a significant part of the diet. In today's marketplace, we have an abundance of high-quality plant protein choices. Soy, because of its versatility and use in many different foods, is one of the most popular, although it is not without its downside. Nonetheless, it is widely used in meat substitutes, dairy substitutes, snack foods, and an endless variety of other products.

In 1999 the Food and Drug Administration issued a statement that including soy in our diets could reduce the risk of heart disease, which was then and still is the number one cause of death in the US. Today soy still enjoys great popularity and is heavily marketed in the form of tofu, edamame, soy cheeses, and soy meats. It is also an additive in many if not most processed foods. Here are some of the reasons that it has become a protein source of choice.

Soy is an excellent source of lean protein, and when used instead of meat, which has a higher fat content, it is a heart-healthy alternative that can aid in weight management, lower triglycerides, and reduce inflammation. There are conflicting studies and opinions about soy as a healthy plant protein. Most stem from the phytoestrogens in soy which can cause the risks associated with too much of this hormone in both men and women. As an example, in some women, soy's phytoestrogens improve menopause symptoms, and in others it makes them worse. The same conflicting results have occurred in cancer studies. In some, soy consumption is linked to lower ovarian and breast cancer risk. Although there have been conflicting conclusions drawn from studies on the risk of breast cancer recurrence, the evidence is now more consistent that soy decreases that risk. It is still unclear whether soy increases or decreases the risk of prostate cancer.

Because the consumption of soy can produce or influence very different health outcomes for individuals, eating it in small to moderate amounts is the key. Organic, non-GMO soy can be a valuable part of a balanced healthy diet, in which a wide variety of whole vegetables, fruits, nuts, and grains are the staples.

Legumes

Other members of the legume family, including beans, peas, and lentils in all their varieties, are staple protein sources in vegetarian and vegan diets, as well as being popular with meat eaters. Because they are relatively inexpensive, they have provided protein for most of the world's populations for centuries. In the US in lower income communities, and certainly in less affluent times for the country as a whole, meat was a luxury. Our current appetite for meat as the centerpiece of most meals developed with the affluence of the

Beans and rice remain a healthy, delicious, cost-effective, and satisfying protein staple for many families and are a personal favorite of mine.

last several decades and the growth and influence of big agriculture with its concentrated factory meat production.

And legumes, whether beans, lentils, garbanzo beans, peas, or a myriad of others, are excellent sources of protein and foods of choice in many parts of the world. When eaten in combination with other carbohydrates—Mexican beans and rice, Indian dal and rice, Japanese soybeans and rice or Cajun red beans and rice—we get the benefit of a plant-based meal containing complete protein with all the necessary amino acids.

HEALTHY CARBS
Whole Grains

Many healthy carbohydrates are also good sources of protein, particularly when eaten in combination with other plant foods. Whole grains like brown, red, or black rice, quinoa, barley, wheat, and rye are delicious and provide protein for growth, development, and maintenance of lean muscle. Organic, non-GMO corn eaten fresh or in the form of polenta, grits, or hominy is also a delicious protein source. Quinoa, sometimes called the king of grains because it is a complete protein source, is native to South America but has gained popularity in the US and worldwide for its healthful properties. It is a good source of calcium, magnesium, potassium, iron, zinc, phosphorous, manganese, and other minerals.

Seeds and Nuts

Seeds, nuts, and nut butters are great protein sources and are best eaten raw and unfiltered for full health benefit of their enzymes and natural, unprocessed healthy fats. One ounce of pumpkin seeds contains 9.35 grams of protein! That's over two grams more than the same quantity of ground beef.[24] Their high protein and nutrient content make them a wonderful addition to any salad or snack.

My favorite breakfast consists of a big plate of whatever fresh and seasonal fruit is in my fridge—oranges, grapefruit, berries, watermelon, apples, grapes—and whole organic flaxseed that I sometimes grind with sprouted pumpkin seeds, raw chia seeds, or raw sesame seeds for a great tasting breakfast. The seeds take less than a minute to grind in my coffee grinder and taste great with a mild nutty flavor that changes with the combinations I choose. My "seed cereal" pairs well with the sweet juicy fruit. It's very filling, and I eat it from a small bowl just like a cereal. To pump up the protein even higher, I often spread raw crunchy almond butter on my apple slices or on a toasted Ezekiel sprouted grain English muffin.

Flaxseed is one of the most powerful antioxidants and is rich in inflammation-fighting, heart-protecting omega-3, lignans, and linoleic acids. Because of its anti-inflammatory properties, it is preferred over fish as a source of omega-3 and is a mainstay for many vegans.

Walnuts are an excellent source of protein, omega-3, and linoleic acid, and are a great heart-healthy food. Almonds are the most protein-rich, nutrient-dense nut, which means they will keep you full longer. With one ounce (approximately 24 nuts) containing 6.03 grams of protein, they are a wonderful addition to any snack or meal. Almonds contain calcium, folic acid, riboflavin, niacin, magnesium, which is also good for heart and muscle health, and other important minerals. Pistachios are delicious, and compared to other nuts, a lower calorie food that can be eaten as a snack or used in the preparation of desserts and salads, or in cooking.

As a personal preference and health choice, although I eat nuts sparingly, I choose raw nuts because I want to enjoy all the nutrients as nature intended, and in particular I want to avoid the effect of heat on the oils they contain. As a rule you will want to avoid nuts that are salted, sugared, flavored, or otherwise processed. The added sugar and salt add empty, not healthy, calories.

HEALTHY FATS VS. PROCESSED OILS

Healthy fats are those that are eaten as part of the plant that produced them—olives, avocados, sesame seeds, almonds, and such. Our bodies need fat, but the FDA guideline of eating 30 percent of your daily calories in fats is very high and based on a diet that includes meat and dairy. To naturally reverse heart disease and help prevent the level of inflammation that promotes other lifestyle diseases, including diabetes, cancer, and Alzheimer's, the maximum fat consumed needs to be closer to 10–15 percent according to some studies on nutritional cures.

The heart disease reversal program I followed with my cardiologist, like the ones developed by Dr. Esselstyn and Dr. Ornish, does not allow any extracted oils to be used on or in foods in their program for their patients whose goal is to reverse heart disease. None. They are adamant about this because of the damage oil does to the epithelial cells that line the blood vessels and arteries. The damage is immediate and causes plaque to form as the lining attempts to heal. It makes sense not to continue the damage during the healing process. *Again, think of the cells working so hard to repair the damage yet we keep pouring oil on, in effect working against ourselves.* Eventually they cannot keep up, and our arteries are clogged, leading to a stent, bypass, or heart attack.

After my symptoms of cardiovascular disease were eliminated, I added a little cold-pressed, extra virgin olive oil back to salad dressings, and ate vegan dishes that sometimes contained processed oil. I also got into a daily habit of eating raw nuts and seeds—walnuts, pistachios, cashews, and Brazil nuts—as snacks because they were tasty, satisfying, and convenient. After a few months, my blood pressure readings started a slow rise. When I looked at the amount of fat I had started consuming daily, I was shocked to see that it was over 50 percent of my total calorie intake, even higher than the FDA guideline and five times the amount that had eliminated my symptoms! Again I listened to my body, stopped using oils, cut back on high fat content foods, and in about three months I was back to normal blood pressure readings.

What I have found is that by eliminating extracted oils in foods, I can enjoy walnuts or other heart-healthy nuts and seeds sparingly, mainly as a topping or ingredient in food without any problem. This was another lesson for me that fat, like sugar, is healthiest when it is eaten as part of the whole food that produced it. I now agree with those who say there is no "healthy oil" extracted product. Without processed oil in cooked foods or on salads, I slowly began to appreciate the natural flavors of the food I once poured it in or on. I now prefer foods without it.

For those who are not reversing disease and are not ready to give up oil, there are oils that are "less unhealthy." The most popular is cold-pressed extra virgin olive oil; however, it is not recommended for cooking because it is not as heat tolerant as grape-seed oil, for example. Many people like coconut oil, which is high in saturated fat, and for that reason can be a problem over time. Limiting the amount of cold-pressed oil added to foods is very important and limiting cooked oils even more so. A good tip for those who use extra virgin olive oil when cooking pasta is to add a little immediately after draining it, toss and let it rest for a few minutes. There will be enough heat to let the pasta absorb the oil but not so much heat as to alter its qualities. Overall use any processed oil sparingly, if at all.

The point of this chapter is that we have many healthy and delicious choices to provide us with both good food and good health. Eating mindfully is not about what we can't eat; it is about an awareness of the abundant food choices we have and making those choices in a way that takes care of our health and supports the health of our families, communities, and planet. It is also about celebrating choice and abundance, while enjoying an endless variety of ways to prepare and enjoy delicious *and* healthy foods.

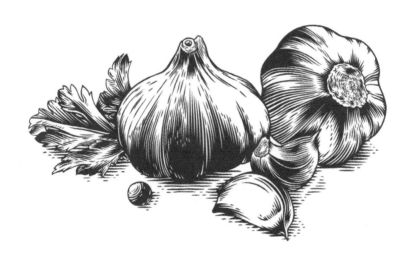

CHAPTER 8

The Spice of Life

"Nature is so smart, it put the medicine inside the food."
—Author unknown

ONE OF THE BEST RULES FOR feeding yourself in a healthy and enjoyable way is to eat a wide variety of foods, prepared in many different ways. This is part of the process of expanding awareness of the bountiful universe in which we live and the infinite number of ways we are nurtured by it. Although some foods are indigenous to a single country or region, most have been adapted to grow in many different areas of the world.

> Often the major difference in the cuisine of one country or region compared to the next is not the food itself, but the method of preparation, including the spice and herb preferences that are part of the culture.

SPICES AND BENEFITS

Many herbs and spices have medicinal properties and have been used for centuries in folk medicine traditions, offering additional options to support our health and healing. Today these are widely available and popular in the US. For example:

- **Cayenne pepper** fights inflammation, helps digestion, is a natural blood thinner, fights clotting, relieves joint/nerve pain, provides detox support, fights bronchial infection, boosts metabolism, and more.
- **Turmeric** contains curcumin, a powerful anti-inflammatory compound shown to be effective in treating arthritis, cancer, Alzheimer's disease, and depression, and lowering risk of heart disease.
- **Cumin (Comino)** aids digestion, relieves respiratory disorders and the common cold, treats insomnia, anemia, skin disorders, and cancer.
- **Ginger** supports digestion, fights inflammation and cancer, lowers blood sugar as an anti-diabetic, relieves menstrual pain, lowers cholesterol, improves heart risk factors, improves brain function, and fights infections.
- **Garlic** contains allicin which supports the digestive tract and stomach lining, fights colds, lowers blood pressure, lowers cholesterol, helps prevent Alzheimer's and dementia, promotes healthy aging, can enhance physical performance (it was given to Olympic athletes in ancient Greece), and may improve bone health. Raw garlic that has been cut or crushed and allowed to sit for about five to ten minutes is more potent than garlic left uncut or garlic that has been cooked.
- **Rosemary** boosts memory, improves mood, reduces inflammation, stimulates circulation, protects against bacterial infections, heals skin conditions, detoxifies the body, soothes the stomach, and aids the immune system.

- **Thyme** stimulates appetite, relieves sore throat, cold symptoms, whooping cough, bronchitis, and colic, soothes upset stomach, relieves gas and diarrhea, treats skin disorders, is a natural diuretic, and treats parasitic worm infections.
- **Mint** clears the palate, stimulates the appetite, supports bronchial function, soothes skin, counters nausea, assists memory, helps with depression, fatigue, and headache, treats asthma, freshens the mouth and breath, aids digestion, and supports weight loss.
- **Curry** contains turmeric, cumin, and cardamom in powder form and therefore has the benefits of those herbs listed above; it also promotes liver function and can decrease pain from inflammation.
- **Oregano** is known for its antifungal properties and antibacterial effects; it is a cancer fighter because of its rich antioxidant content, which protects cells and helps fight infection; some research suggests that oil of a Himalayan oregano may kill the hospital super-bug MRSA, and it is potent even when boiled; it is also used to treat headache, fatigue, and respiratory problems.
- **Sage** contains rosmarinic acid, a potent antioxidant as well as an anti-inflammatory agent useful in treating rheumatoid arthritis, bronchial asthma, and atherosclerosis; aids memory and brain function, and has potential for treating Alzheimer's; has been used for hot flashes and menopause symptoms.
- **Bay Leaf** extract is used in aromatherapy and for the treatment of some respiratory and skin conditions; can be used as a diuretic and is helpful for upset stomach, irritable bowel syndrome, and lessening celiac disease symptoms; has natural antibacterial properties.
- **Cardamom** is related to ginger and has similar benefits: it aids digestion; helps with constipation, bloating, and loss of appetite; treats mouth ulcers, bad breath, and depression; provides

antispasmodic treatment for hiccups; supports kidneys through detox and diuretic properties; lowers blood pressure; and inhibits bacteria and virus growth. The ancients considered it an aphrodisiac!

PEPPERS

Researchers have discovered that capsaicin, the compound that gives jalapeños, habaneros, and cayenne chili peppers a powerful kick, can help burn more calories immediately after a meal. Black pepper and ginger have similar effects. Chipotle peppers are dried and smoked jalapeños, but because of their smoky and slightly sweet taste, the hot flavor may appear somewhat softer. Drying chipotle peppers removes some of the heat, which makes it easier to add this spice to your foods. The flavor and benefits make it popular with health-conscious chefs and home cooks alike.

If you can enjoy or can tolerate them, peppers in general help reduce cholesterol, triglyceride levels, and platelet aggregation; they also help increase your body's ability to dissolve fibrin, a substance known to form blood clots. And they lower free radical damage that leads to the development of atherosclerosis. Weight control is easier with improvements to circulation and metabolism. The chemical compounds in chipotle can dilate blood vessels, improving circulation and reducing the risk of heart disease. [25]

The BBC News has stated that capsaicin in jalapeños also instigates cancer cell suicide, known scientifically as apoptosis. In a study at Nottingham University in the UK, scientists tested the capsaicin on both lung and pancreatic cancer cells and found that it triggered cell suicide. Because of the capsaicin levels, chipotle, habanero, and cayenne peppers help to stop prostate cancer cells from spreading and can help prostate cancer tumors to shrink in size.

The capsaicin in chipotle and other hot peppers also helps reduce the risk of type 2 diabetes. It both affects the production of insulin and increases the rate at which the liver clears the insulin. As mentioned before, capsaicin also aids fat oxidization, which leads to increased weight loss. Since the development of type 2 diabetes goes hand and hand with obesity, this is another way that chipotle can help reduce the risk of that disease as well.

These and other herbs and spices are used to enhance the flavor of many dishes, promote overall health, and generally have no negative side effects in the small amounts normally used in food preparation. To achieve the specific health benefits noted above, some may have to be taken in a concentrated form as a dietary supplement, in which case you must consult with your health care provider for the appropriate dosage. Remember that herbs can interact with medicines you take and make them either more or less effective, so in this case, your physician's advice should guide you.

There are three points to be made here. First, there are an unlimited number of ways to prepare traditional foods creatively if we take the time to try new things and be just a little adventurous.

Second, it's important to note that the beneficial properties of the small sampling of herbs and spices presented here often overlap. In other words, these herbs and spices enhance and complement each other, and when eaten with vegetables, legumes, and grains, there are cumulative and interactive effects that no study can measure. *In real life, we eat foods in combinations, which adds power to their healing effects.*

Third, we can, as part of learning to eat mindfully, select and add herbs and spices to our everyday meals with thought as to how our body may benefit from them. And just as importantly, if while we enjoy good health, we develop this habit of feeding ourselves consciously—by adding these ingredients to fresh, whole foods—we may reduce or eliminate the need for drugs to maintain good health for many years. And many of us may never have to rely on them!

RESURGENCE OF NUTRITIONAL MEDICINE

Humans relied for thousands of years on herbal medicines to enhance health and treat illnesses. The ancient Egyptians produced a listing of over eight hundred medicinal herbs, which includes many that are still used today, and in the US in the late 1800s, the practice of herbal medicine flourished and was taught in medical schools and universities. This changed with the formation of the American Medical Association (AMA) in 1848 by the advocates of the scientific method, spurred by the rise of American industry, the successful development of vaccines and antibiotics, and the general belief that science and manufacturing would solve all problems. What is little known is that John D. Rockefeller saw an opportunity to create a new medical industry based on the manufacture of pharmaceuticals and the training of medical students in drug therapies and surgical procedures. By 1935 more than half of all American medical schools had either closed or merged with large universities. Standardization of medical training was established by the AMA, and schools that offered naturopathic, herbal, or other such courses were forced to drop them or lose accreditation.[26]

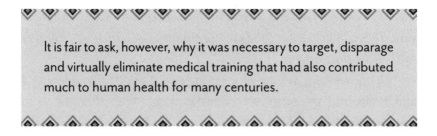

It is fair to ask, however, why it was necessary to target, disparage and virtually eliminate medical training that had also contributed much to human health for many centuries.

So here we are, a hundred years later, with epidemic public health crises of diabetes, heart disease, obesity, and cancer, while our medical establishment still approaches health care from a mindset formed in the industrial revolution. To be sure, the advances of drugs such as antibiotics and vaccines against diseases like polio have been invaluable and have saved countless lives.

◇◇◇◇◇◇◇◇◇◇◇◇◇

It is troubling that the profit motive to create and control a new industry was so influential in bringing us to this point where we have declining health and skyrocketing drug costs. How much better off would we be if collaboration, or at least mutual respect for the best of both the medical worlds, had been allowed to evolve?

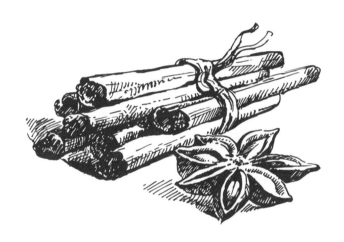

CHAPTER 9

World of Flavor:
Regional and International

"Food is our common ground, a universal experience."
—James Beard

BY TRYING A WIDE VARIETY OF foods prepared in healthful combinations with different spices, we learn to delight our palates and discover how foods, spices, and herbs can be healing as well as delicious. In doing so, we learn to appreciate the healing foods offered up by Mother Earth and used in culinary traditions around the world. Here are some favorites that can spice up our healthy food creativity.

AMERICAN SOUL FOOD
Most of us continue to eat the same foods, prepared in the same way that our parents and grandparents did. We do this even though many of the conditions that shaped their diet have changed or even

> The only limits to our enjoyment of the foods we eat are those we put on our imagination and our willingness to try new experiences.

vanished entirely. A case in point: I grew up in the South, where vegetables boiled with salt pork, fat back, or other fatty meat for flavor are still a dietary staple. Few people ever stop to think about the reason for this Southern food tradition. One theory is that in the rural American south in the seventeenth and eighteenth centuries, most people had no choice but to eat what they produced. There was limited availability of the condiments and spices to which we now have ready access. If this was true for the general population, it was even more so for the slaves whose descendants perfected dishes of collard greens, black-eyed peas, and turnips seasoned with what they had available—salted pork which was cured or smoked to preserve it without refrigeration. These are still signature "soul food" dishes. They have been handed down from generation to generation and are still prepared exactly the same way. And those of you who have had them know they are really tasty.

Here is the point. We now know several things that were not widely known in the rural South of the 1800s when our great-great-grandparents used the foods and cooking methods available to them to create a cuisine that is still celebrated today for its great taste and lasting appeal:

- Excess salt and fat are not healthy.
- Boiling or otherwise overcooking vegetables destroys the enzymes which enable us to assimilate the nutrients they contain and destroys many nutrients as well.
- Combining other vegetables and spices such as garlic, onion, cumin, and celery in fresh or condiment form can

produce the same flavors as pork, beef, or chicken, or even more interesting and varied ones.

In recent years significant numbers of people like me, raised in this tradition, are using our twenty-first-century nutritional knowledge and a wide variety of readily available produce and spices to recreate these dishes in equally delicious, yet healthier ways. Cooking time for greens like collards has been cut to twenty minutes or less from several hours, and some people now add a leaner smoked turkey leg instead of pork fat. Others have eliminated the meat altogether and steam or sauté collard or turnip greens with spices for even a shorter time to achieve the same taste in much healthier versions. In the recipe section of this book, you will find other soul food favorites healthily reimagined!

ASIAN

Asian cooking can be quick, tasty, and healthy. Vegetables and even seafood, for those who choose to eat it, can be stir fried in a matter of minutes. Some ingredients are grown locally, and others like ginger and water chestnuts are likely not. Most, including bok choy, snow peas, eggplant, scallions, peppers, mushrooms, mustard greens, and celery, are available at your local supermarket. You can choose the Earth friendly solution and substitute local produce for ingredients not locally produced. Flexibility and creativity are the key.

Asian spice blends are known for providing the perfect balance of aromatic, hot, savory, sour, and sweet sensations to each meal. The spices that are typically used in Asian cuisine are basil, cinnamon, cilantro, coriander, chiles, cloves, cumin, garlic, ginger, lemongrass, spearmint, star anise, and turmeric. Fresh leafy spices also play an important role in garnishing plates and include basil, cilantro, lemongrass, mint, and scallions. Other condiments commonly used in Asian-inspired recipes include tamari, curry, and horseradish.

Many Asian dishes are easy to adapt to a vegan version by substituting tofu or a plant-based meat like seitan or tempeh. Seitan is made from wheat gluten, and unless you are gluten sensitive, it is a very satisfying and versatile meat substitute that can be grilled, sautéed, or baked. It can be flavored with herbs and spices to taste like chicken, beef, pork, or fish. It is available in many grocery stores in a variety of flavors. Tempeh is made from fermented soybeans and is more textured and firmer than tofu, which makes it a good substitute for fish or ground beef. Like seitan, it can be flavored in many ways, depending on the dish you want to use it in, and it is also found in most supermarkets. Although these can be incredibly delicious meat substitutes, they are processed foods with added ingredients like oils, soy sauce, or liquid aminos. So read the label to manage your salt and fat intake when you use them, and to make sure there are no ingredients that you want to avoid, the standing rule with any packaged food.

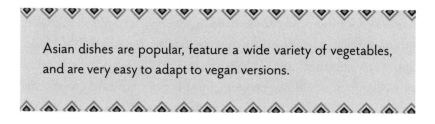

Asian dishes are popular, feature a wide variety of vegetables, and are very easy to adapt to vegan versions.

⋄⋄⋄⋄⋄⋄⋄⋄⋄⋄⋄⋄

Please check out the cookbooks included in the resource section of this book for plenty of recipes and inspiration!

AFRICAN

African cuisine is less familiar to most of us in the US and varies widely based on the country of origin. My husband was born in Senegal in West Africa, so I am most familiar with the food traditions of that region. The basic Senegalese diet is based on flavored rice served with a medley of vegetables. Fish, lamb, or chicken is usually added and served with several side sauces to complement the particular dish. Senegalese cooking is a wonderful fusion of West African cuisine with French culinary influences. Fish and meats are often infused with spice and herb mixtures that enhance their taste. Sauces are intricately layered with flavor upon flavor. The result is a culinary tradition with many healthy attributes that can be easily adapted to further enhance its healthful qualities. I have included a couple of Senegalese recipes, simplified and adapted to reduce preparation time while retaining the wonderful flavors. First is my vegan gumbo, a flavorful version of the Senegalese soupe kandia which I love to make and to eat!

The national dish of Senegal is thieboudienne. Although fish or meat adds additional flavor, these dishes are delightfully tasty with or without animal protein. The trick to achieving a meat, fish, or chicken flavor in a vegan dish is through the use of spice and texture combinations in the recipe. Another healthy adaptation of Senegalese cooking is the substitution of organic brown rice for white. Finally, since much of the flavor is in the sauce, Senegalese cooks often cook the vegetables in the sauce over time until the flavors blend. This means that much of the enzyme and nutritional content of the vegetables is lost. *To reduce this loss and maintain the vibrant colors and textures of the vegetables, I've learned to use a little bit of each vegetable to make a flavorful sauce that is simmered as a base to produce the rich blended flavor.* Then I add to the sauce the fresh vegetables that need only ten or fifteen minutes cooking time, quickly followed by those like cauliflower that need five minutes or less. The entire vegetable stew can then rest away from the heat to allow the latest additions to absorb the wonderful flavors of the base before serving.

Some of the spices, herbs, and oils producing West African cuisine's delightful flavors include paprika, red pepper, garlic, curry, mustard, red palm oil, and tamarind. Vegetables include tomatoes, onions, celery, peppers, eggplant, cabbage, carrots, and cauliflower, potatoes, and yucca root, which is one of my favorites. I hope you will try the vegan version of thieboudienne, the national dish of Senegal. Enjoy!

INDIAN

Indian cuisine is renowned for its vegetarian traditions coupled with a cornucopia of spices to delight the senses. Although some dishes are made with milk or yogurt to "cool the fire," most can be adapted to suit a vegan diet. The spices commonly used in Indian cuisine include curry powder, cumin, nutmeg, mustard seeds, red pepper, ginger, and cloves. Cloves, which have a very distinct taste and fragrance, must be used sparingly so as not to overpower other more subtle herbs and spices. The clove is actually a flower whose fragrance comes primarily from the oils it contains, and it has been used in traditional healing for centuries. It has active antioxidant, local anesthetic, stomach soothing, anti-gas, and anti-constipation properties. Cloves also contain essential oils that give them a pleasant aromatic fragrance and a warming and soothing quality along with their medicinal benefits.

Mustard seeds, which are related to cruciferous plants like broccoli, Brussels sprouts, and cabbage, contain a powerhouse of nutritional benefits just like their cousins. These include phytonutrients and enzymes, which studies have shown to have an anti-cancer effect that inhibits the formation and growth of cancer cells in the colon and the gastrointestinal tract. The anti-inflammatory effects of the selenium and magnesium in mustard seeds are additional benefits of eating this spice. Selenium is a nutrient that can reduce the effects of asthma, rheumatoid arthritis, and cancer. The magnesium in mustard seeds can help restore normal sleep patterns, reduce migraine frequency, lower high blood pressure, and prevent heart attacks in patients with atherosclerosis or diabetic heart disease. They are also a good source of omega-3, omega-6, protein, calcium, and vitamin B-1.

Nutmeg is an aromatic and slightly sweet spice used a lot in Indian cooking. It has a long list of associated health benefits, including its ability to relieve pain, soothe indigestion, strengthen cognitive function, detoxify the body, boost skin health, alleviate oral conditions, reduce insomnia, increase immune system function, prevent leukemia, and improve blood circulation.

Garam marsala, a popular Indian spice combination, includes varying combinations of several of the following ingredients: cloves, turmeric, paprika, salt, cinnamon, garlic, ginger, fennel, cardamom, peppercorns, coriander, and star anise. Indian cuisine is truly rich in healthy, savory spices with many beneficial properties. Please try the savory oil-free Indian vegetable curry in the recipe section.

SOUTHWEST–MEXICAN

Southwest and Mexican dishes are another favorite of mine. The flavors are rich and distinctive and include as ingredients many of the foods I love the most: onion, tomatoes, avocados, green chiles, cilantro, beans, corn, and potatoes. I can always visit one of my favorite Mexican restaurants on one of my all-raw days and enjoy guacamole with pico de gallo, along with a salad or, better yet, a salad with avocado and pico de gallo included. Pico can also be added to beans, black-eyed peas, soups, or even sprinkled on a veggie burger to add extra flavor and a little kick! It's super easy to make, and you'll find it in the recipe section.

Another favorite is tortilla soup made with vegetables, topped with toasted corn tortilla strips, and tasty without the chicken stock commonly used. The spices frequently used in this dish and in most Mexican and Southwest cooking include cumin (comino), paprika, chile powder, garlic, chipotle, and cilantro. To make a vegan version of Mexican tortilla soup, just substitute vegetable broth for the chicken stock.

Cilantro is actually the leaf of the coriander plant. It is packed with antioxidants, essential oils, fiber, and vitamins. It's also a good source of minerals like manganese, phosphorous, calcium, potassium, and iron. Potassium helps regulate blood pressure and heart rate. It is rich in vitamins A and C and is one of the richest herbal sources of vitamin K, which plays a role in promoting bone health and has been demonstrated to help limit neuron brain damage in Alzheimer's disease patients.

Paprika is a powdered spice made from dried bell peppers and chili peppers. One tablespoon provides 100 percent of the recommended dietary allowance (RDA) of vitamin A, which improves night vision. It is rich in carotenoids, the pigments in paprika that give it its deep red color and protect the eyes. Paprika also boosts your daily intake of vitamin E. Each tablespoon provides 2 milligrams of vitamin E, or 13 percent of the recommended daily intake determined by the Institute of Medicine. Vitamin E helps control blood clot formation and promotes healthy blood vessel function. Getting enough vitamin E in your diet also promotes healthy cell communication, or cellular coherence, as I like to think of it. In other words, it helps our trillions of cells share information and operate in harmony.

My Mexican spinach salad recipe, made with ingredients I combed through a steakhouse menu to find, is so good that I've started making it at home. Some of my favorite dishes were improvised from restaurant menus lacking vegetarian or vegan options, but with lots of salad and side order options to repurpose as entrées!

ITALIAN

You may remember my story about being lost and hungry at night on a highway outside of Tulsa, and after almost settling for a veggie Subway, enjoying a memorable vegan Italian-style meal made by a creative young chef at my hotel! The Mediterranean diet is renowned for several healthy attributes, and with a little tweaking it can be even more so, without sacrificing flavor or enjoyment. First the spices: garlic (used for centuries as a healing food), basil, parsley, oregano, pepperoncino (hot chili pepper), bay leaves, sage, rosemary, and thyme are the staples.

We usually think of pasta when we think of Italian food. Although whole wheat pastas are somewhat healthier than the conventional semolina wheat pastas, let's face it . . . it's still a processed food, so I advise eating it sparingly. For those times when you choose to enjoy it, I recommend some other varieties of pasta made from high protein, gluten-free whole grains. One of those is pasta made from quinoa, which cooks in about the same time as whole wheat pasta but remains al dente or firm with a more substantial texture. I also enjoy brown rice pastas, which are gluten free and made with whole brown rice grains for texture and fiber.

I like to sauté onion and garlic with other ingredients and a little water to create a pasta sauce rather than using oil. If you must use oil for a traditional sauté, try grape-seed or almond, which hold up well under heat. As mentioned in chapter 7, olive oil is not high heat tolerant and changes composition in the process of cooking, losing some of its desirable properties, although I may use a bit—extra virgin and cold pressed—to top off a dish for flavor after cooking, for dipping, or to dress a salad. Increasingly, I find myself eliminating the oil, as I have grown to enjoy dishes better without it.

What's the next thing we think of when we think Italian? Why pizza, of course! Although it's debated as to whether pizza actually originated in Italy, the reputation stuck. One of my favorite vegan restaurants is a little eatery on Sunset Boulevard in Los Angeles about three blocks from my daughter, who lives in Silver Lake. Now when we plan a trip to see her family or my daughter and family in Glassel Park, I get excited, first about spending time with all of them, and second about having the killer vegan pizza at Flore Vegan. The crust is made from corn meal that, when baked, is the right texture mix between crispy and chewy and holds up very well under the house-made tomato sauce. The cheese, ah, the cheese is house-made from cashews, and although the consistency is lighter than mozzarella or other dairy cheeses, the taste is delicate, delicious, and, well . . . cheesy. It's topped with your choice of fresh organic vegetables, much like any other pizza, and then oven baked. Cashew cheese is easy to make, and the recipe is included. If you don't want to make your own vegan cheese at home, Gaia is the best I've found in the supermarket.

Granted the very thought of having a really good vegan pizza is exciting enough. And this is pretty damn good pizza. You can find some good vegan pizza choices in the frozen food section of most supermarkets. Remember to read the ingredient list and nutrition facts on the box.

MIDDLE EASTERN

With a similar array of spices as Indian cuisine, but with unique flavors and some distinct preparation methods, Middle Eastern cuisine is savory, exotic for the Western palate, and fascinating. Although Middle Eastern and Northern African cuisines incorporate lamb, chicken, beef, and fish as an important component of many dishes, it adapts easily to vegetarian and vegan versions.

Hummus, one of the staples of vegetarian and vegan fare, is easy to make and rich in protein. The basic ingredient is garbanzo beans, which are blended with lemon juice, tahini, garlic, and spices, and can be made with or without olive oil. It can be flavored by adding other ingredients such as red pepper, chipotle, spinach, and the like.

You can find many varieties of hummus in your local supermarket. It's great as a spread or a dip for a quick, healthy snack, and so tasty. It's delicious, easy to make, and there are vegan recipes by the dozen on the internet.

Another healthy Middle Eastern treat is tabouli, a healthy, tasty mixture of chopped parsley, bulgur, onion, tomato, and spices. For the slightly more adventurous, Moroccan tagine cooking is very interesting and seals in the food flavors. A tagine is a conical shaped earthenware dish with a cone-shaped top that fits snugly inside the base. According to some sources, it dates back to an eighth-century BC ruler of the Islamic empire, but certainly was popularized by the Berber people who were early inhabitants of this North African country. I like to think of it as the original crock pot, made from clay to slow cook over hot coals. Its cone shape captures the steam rising from the cooking food and allows it to condense and trickle back down into the food itself. This intensifies the flavor of the food because little water is required in the process. The word tagine also refers to the food cooked in this manner, which is flavorful with spice combinations and has come to define a distinctly Moroccan taste. Just enter "Moroccan vegan recipes" in your browser, and you'll be surprised by how many you'll find to try.

◇◇◇◇◇◇◇◇◇◇◇◇◇

I hope this little trip through a few major culinary traditions from various parts of the globe reinforces the idea that you can find healthy and enjoyable food wherever you are. As a conscious eater, part of the enjoyment of food is learning more about the culture that produced it, along with traditional ingredients and preparation. From there we can tweak ingredients, preparation methods, or both, if necessary, for a healthier dish, while preserving the flavors, textures, and overall experience. Broadening our food horizons adds variety and excitement to healthy eating and helps us experience the tastes and health benefits of new plants, herbs, spices, and preparation methods.

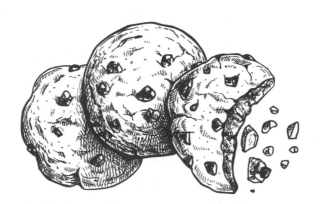

CHAPTER 10

For Your Sweet Tooth

"Food for the body is not enough. There must be food for the soul."

—DOROTHY DAY

OKAY, I ADMIT IT. I definitely have a sweet tooth. We saw in the chapter on food addictions how naturally occurring sugars helped early humans to survive and evolve. As a result, we are hard-wired to like sugar and, of course, as with anything, some of us like it more than others . . . and I'm probably on the "like it more" side. I shared how, as a kid, the best part of any birthday was the cake, and the best part of the cake was the icing! I also learned at six years old how to make my own hot cocoa on the gas stove. If we were out of Nestle's Quick I would make my own chocolate syrup from Hershey's Cocoa, sugar, and milk—and I was in heaven. And, of course, every time I earned money for chores, at least part of it went with me to the neighborhood grocer to buy a Tootsie Roll, moon cookies, Hostess CupCakes, or a soda. I hope you can see why I am so grateful for the good health that I enjoy! My cells have given me countless do-overs while holding up under a small mountain of sugar over time.

What my parents, like most Americans, failed to realize at the time was that a diet high in sugar presents long-term health hazards far beyond simple weight gain, cavities, and even the risk of diabetes. Although information is now widely available about how processed cane sugar, high-fructose corn syrup, and overuse of concentrated natural sugars in the form of fruit juices or syrups play a key role in diabetes, heart disease, and some cancers, we still find it difficult to avoid too much sugar in our diet. This is especially true if we eat processed foods. Most of us, myself included, have to pay attention to how much sugar we eat, and to try and get most of that sugar by eating whole fruit.

Is it possible to have your cake and eat it too, figuratively speaking? I say yes by being selective about the sweeteners and other ingredients we use in sweet treats, not eating them daily, and eating only small portions. And we can limit the impact of the sugar we consume with good old-fashioned moderation. *Diabetics and those of us who may be prediabetic will have to exercise special caution and consult with a health care provider about the suitability of any desserts including the ones presented here.*

Smoothies, which I talked about in chapter 6 under raw foods, make great sweet treats. Using the whole fruit means that the fiber will work against blood sugar spikes. They are ridiculously easy to make and hard to get wrong. When the fruit is in season, local, and naturally ripened, almost any combination will be sweet and delicious. And to ramp up the nutritional value, add one or two vegetables to the mix like kale, spinach, carrots, or beets. Just throw it in the blender with some ice, and there you go.

PLANT-BASED BAKING TIPS

If you haven't tried plant-based bakery and pastry items, you are in for a very pleasant surprise. Most cakes, cookies, and other desserts are naturally plant based, except for the eggs, butter, and milk. These ingredients have simple, healthy substitution options that will not usually change the taste or texture of the final product. Most people cannot tell the difference! And the following substitutions will deliver more nutritional value with less inflammation for your body.

Egg Substitutes

Although there are egg substitute products sold in supermarkets, the best ones I've found are simple, natural, and do a very good job as a binding agent. This is basically the function that eggs perform in holding cakes or other baked goods together. My go-to product is flax seed, which I keep in my refrigerator for freshness and grind when I'm ready to use it.

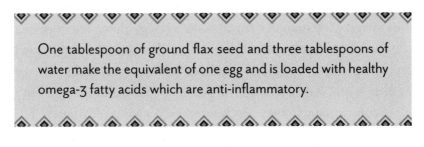

One tablespoon of ground flax seed and three tablespoons of water make the equivalent of one egg and is loaded with healthy omega-3 fatty acids which are anti-inflammatory.

Mix and let stand for three to five minutes, and it is ready to use as you would egg in your recipe. The other ingredient used as a substitute for eggs in many baked goods is good old-fashioned, unsweetened applesauce, which is also an excellent binding agent.

Plant Milks

This is easy-peasy. Just choose from the many plant milks available: oat, almond, hemp, soy, rice, and the like. Choose your favorite and keep it on hand. These are all available off the shelf and don't need refrigeration until after they are opened. Some have vanilla flavoring and are sweetened, so choose carefully. There are so many brands in stores that we also have the opportunity to buy from companies that are committed to our health and the environment, so read the labels! And of course you can make your own milk. My favorite is hemp milk and there is a recipe for making it in the recipe section. It takes only five minutes!

Cobblers and Cookies

A very easy dessert that can be made in a healthful way without sacrificing taste is the fruit cobbler. By swapping out some traditional ingredients in favor of healthier and equally tasty ones, this dessert scores in both the health and taste columns. If the fruit is in season and ripe, an added sweetener won't be necessary. If desired, as shown in the recipe section, a little maple syrup can be substituted for refined sugar. I used almond butter and organic rolled oats mixed with almond flour to make a crispy gluten-free topping.

Fresh apples, peaches, or berries are the most commonly used fruits in crisps or cobblers, and I really like pear cobbler. Or try pairing fruits for an interesting twist . . . how about apple with blueberry or mango with peach or whatever suits your fancy? For an extra treat, sprinkle heart-healthy unsalted raw walnuts on top after it comes out of the oven or add some to the oat–flour mixture before baking.

And don't forget to try the cookie and other vegan dessert recipes in the cookbook references found in the resources section, especially my all-time favorite Oatmeal Raisin Chocolate Chip cookies in the *Engine 2 Cookbook*.

RAW SWEET TREATS
Vegan Ice Creams and Sorbets

It's easier than you may think to find desserts that are incredibly delicious and also check your boxes for healthier treats. Vegan ice creams are a great example. Several brands can be found in many supermarkets that are particularly creamy and good, as well as non-dairy and refined sugar free. Unlike soy or rice milk frozen desserts, coconut milk ice cream is really creamy. It comes in delicious flavors including pomegranate, chocolate chip, mango, German chocolate, vanilla, of course, and many more.

It should come as no surprise that the best vegan ice creams are the ones made fresh in health-conscious eateries or at home in your own kitchen using fresh, raw, organic ingredients like coconuts, almonds, fruit, or raw cacao powder. Vegan ice creams and sorbets can be sweetened with fruit, dates, or other minimally processed or unprocessed sweeteners. Or you can add a little almond, coconut, hemp, or other non-dairy milk with some fresh fruit to make fruity ice cream shakes. It's quick and easy.

Raw Hemp "Milk" Shake

One of the healthiest sweet treats to make at home is a raw hemp milkshake, my favorite. It is one of the creamiest and tastiest seed or nut milks, so good and so easy! Just put a cup of raw shelled hempseeds, three cups of water, dates for sweetness, vanilla to taste and a dash of sea salt in your blender. To achieve the thick creaminess and texture of a traditional milkshake, I don't strain the mixture; if you want a creamy delicious iced milk, just add more water. Add raw cacao or fruit with the other ingredients to create delicious and highly nutritious shakes, super rich in omega-3 fats and antioxidants.

My top healthy dessert pick is the quickest, simplest, and arguably the most decadent of all, and it's all raw. Nuts did you say? How did you know? I take a small handful of my favorite fresh nuts, usually raw almonds, or walnuts, both of which are heart healthy, put them in a dessert cup, and then drizzle them with a little raw honey. The only thing you need to add is a spoon.

There are many resources available for simple and delicious recipes to keep conscious, healthy eating fun and indulgent, including one for a really good vegan cheesecake included in the recipe section.

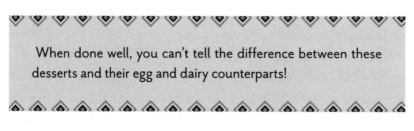

When done well, you can't tell the difference between these desserts and their egg and dairy counterparts!

With your own creativity and the variety of seasonal ingredients available throughout the year, there is no limit. They are so good that you will have to remember the moderation!

CHAPTER 11

Eating and Living Mindfully

"Nothing will benefit health or increase the chances of survival on Earth as the evolution to a vegetarian diet."
—ALBERT EINSTEIN, physicist, 1954

I HOPE THAT YOU ARE ENCOURAGED to begin or continue your journey to improved health with the power of the food and lifestyle changes shared here. Food is our most powerful ally in maintaining or achieving vibrancy, energy, and freedom from pain and from many common diseases. It is our best ally and protector from succumbing to seasonal viruses by keeping our immune system strong. We have the opportunity to make choices every day that will help determine how long we live, the amount of joy we experience, and the quality of our life.

In addition to what we eat, we also know that our emotions and outlook affect our health and ability to prevent or recover from illness. Many leading hospitals and medical facilities are starting to provide spaces for meditation, yoga, and even contact with pets because of the positive effects of these activities on patient recovery.

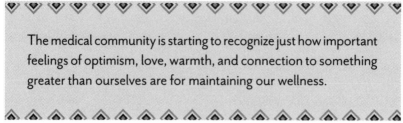

The medical community is starting to recognize just how important feelings of optimism, love, warmth, and connection to something greater than ourselves are for maintaining our wellness.

In chapter 3, I shared a love story that I first heard years ago and that has forever shaped how I appreciate and care for my own health. It focused my attention in a very personal and moving way on the constant devotion our cells lavish on us. From the time we are conceived, our trillions of cells are hard at work using their innate intelligence to promote our growth, health, and longevity. We don't see them doing their work, nor do we really understand how they work, so we take it all for granted. We are not conscious of the critical importance of what they do for us every moment of every day throughout our lives. In addition to this internal energy system that enables our bodies to function, we are part of and supported by nature's larger ecosystem. Nature is more nurturing and intelligent than we ever imagined.

The greatest potential to improve our health lies in our ability to marry health sciences with ancient wisdom and the intelligence of the natural world, including its intangible and spiritual components. We must begin from a place of respect for what we do not know and a commitment to learn from traditional wisdom, nature-centered healing practices, and spiritual traditions that value life in all its forms as an extension of our own. This shift in our thinking and approach will strengthen our ability to sustain good health even as we age. It will also begin to reverse the rising tide of illness and disease with a broader, more holistic approach to health and a primary emphasis on supporting self-care.

This is already beginning to happen. Physicians like Dr. Joel

Fuhrmann, Dr. Dean Ornish, Dr. Neal Barnard, and many others are speaking publicly about our inability to reverse our public health crises without addressing the impact of food, social, and environmental issues. The recognition that we need an integrated approach is highlighted by the rising cost of healthcare while Americans get sicker and sicker. The fragile state of our current medical system has been dramatically exposed by the COVID-19 pandemic.

Preventable lifestyle diseases—heart disease, diabetes, cancer, and dementia—have become our greatest killers, and, as we have learned, increase the threat of the pandemic. Our food system contributes to deforestation, depletion of our protective ozone layer, and pollution of our rivers and air. We are only beginning to see the effects of the resulting climate change which, if our behavior persists, will be disastrous for coastal and inland areas around the globe, and cause major social and economic disruption for all and greater food insecurity for most. *Change will come because we do something significant collectively and individually to change the path we are on, or it will come in a more drastic way if we don't.* We have the ability to help shape and influence our personal and shared destiny.

Our health and survival depend on the natural environment that sustains us. By creating the space to contemplate, meditate, or simply spend time away from daily activity—perhaps in a forest, by a river, at a local farm, or planting tomatoes in your backyard—we allow the simplicity of life to speak for itself. Its message needs no words. In doing so, we slow down, reconnect with what is important, and allow our lives to reflect the simplicity we see in nature. Decisions get easier, thought becomes clearer, we spend more time on things that matter, life becomes fuller and more joyful, and our health thrives. Over time, I have developed an intense, ever present feeling of wonder, appreciation, and compassion for my own physical body—every cell, breath, and heartbeat. It is this real, heartfelt love that fuels and sustains my commitment to feeding myself healthy, beautiful, and delicious food based on what it tells me it needs.

To make the point, compare the recital of a thirty-second grace before a meal to a process that begins by honoring the source of the food and includes the acts of choosing, preparing, and enjoying the entire meal as a continuous expression of gratitude, love, and pleasure. When we are mindful of our connection with all of life, we are more sensitive to our own needs, and our physical, emotional, and spiritual health are enhanced. We move through our daily lives with a sense of self-love, compassion for others, grace, creativity, and joy.

BE THE CHANGE

For those readers who find the idea that listening to your body is the most important aspect of health or that food is the primary cause or cure for most chronic diseases too simplistic, that is actually good news. This book is a call to anyone concerned about their own health to know that a positive, even life-altering impact on the quality of their life is in fact within their reach. By empowering ourselves with the knowledge that our food is indeed our best medicine, we can take responsibility for our health and transform the process of feeding ourselves into a celebration of life. We make this shift, first for ourselves and then to impact those around us, as they observe that there is a practical and powerful way of taking care of ourselves that is healthy, loving, pleasurable, and healing for our planet. As we vote with our forks and our wallets, we also contribute to a much-needed change in our food culture, as we have seen with the explosion in the market for organic and plant-based foods, now the fastest growing segments of the food industry.

HEALTHY YOU, HEALTHY WORLD

There are many healthy food traditions all over the world from which we can learn. The one thing I tried *not* to do in this book is to say that there is only one healthy way to eat. Although we benefit when we eat a diet that consists primarily of whole plant foods, there are healthy meat eaters, and strict vegetarian, vegan, or raw food diets are not necessary for everyone. There are areas in the world where small-scale farming still provides a quality of life for food animals that is respectful of their physical needs and wellbeing. They are fed a natural and chemical-free diet, enjoy fresh air, sunshine, and companionship, and are slaughtered in a humane manner.

As we choose whole plant foods to improve our own personal health, we also reduce needless animal suffering and stop an important source of environmental harm caused by mass production, factory farming of food animals. Perhaps most importantly, we open our minds and hearts to less violent and more compassionate, sustainable ways of living. We desperately need all of these things to occur in order to survive and thrive.

Change always starts with the few and eventually is embraced by the many. Be encouraged to explore the power that is yours to create a healthy and vibrant body, mind, and world. Start wherever you like—by eating more fruits and vegetables, buying organic and non-GMO foods when affordable, shopping at your local farmers' market, joining a food co-op, finding quick, delicious, healthy recipes you love, and supporting with your dollars restaurants and food providers that value your health through the foods they sell. You don't have to do it all, and certainly not all at once. The key is to start—and see where your journey takes you. Remember that every little thing you do along the way counts, even when you don't immediately see or feel the result. It will come, sometimes quickly, but sometimes it takes time. In the same way our tiny cells during our lifetime work hard for years or even decades to limit the impact of the harm we do to ourselves, we have to give them time and good self-care to reverse the damage. As we reap the benefits of good health, our actions will positively impact those around us, our family members, friends, and community. We will offer an example to our children and grandchildren of how to take care of what is most important: good health, good food, clean air and water, a mindful appreciation for the wonder of life, and the joy of living it fully.

recipes

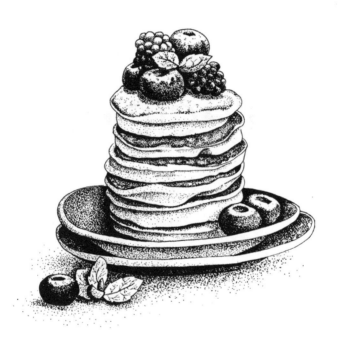

1. BUCKWHEAT PANCAKES

¾ c buckwheat flour

¼ c oat flour (makes fluffier pancakes than all buckwheat)

½ tsp baking powder

½ tsp baking soda

1 pinch salt

2 tbs maple syrup or to taste

1 tbs almond butter

1 tbs vanilla or to taste

¾ c plant-based milk or more for thinner pancakes

1 tbs fresh lemon or lime juice

Optional: blueberries, thin banana, or strawberry slices to press lightly into pancakes before flipping.

Mix dry ingredients in a bowl. In another bowl, mix wet ingredients. Add more plant milk or water for desired thickness. Heat nonstick pan (no oil needed). Flip pancakes after little bubbles form and burst. Keep warm in oven until served.

2. CREAMY RAW HEMP MILK

½ c raw organic hemp seeds

3 c cold water

4 or 5 pitted dates to taste

2 tbs vanilla

1 pinch sea salt

dash of cinnamon (optional)

Add all ingredients and blend in a high-speed blender for 2–3 minutes, or until mixture is smooth. To make a creamy chocolate milk just add 3 heaping tablespoons of raw cacao. Makes 1 quart.

3. ALI'S GREEN SMOOTHIE

1 fresh pineapple
1 bunch fresh parsley
1 whole lemon, unpeeled, quartered and seeds removed
2–3 cloves fresh garlic
1-inch piece of peeled, fresh ginger (or more to taste)
1 c water (or more for desired consistency)
1 tsp raw honey (optional)
1 handful of kale or spinach (optional)

Rinse pineapple, remove top and 1 inch off the bottom, and skin. Rinse again and cut into quarters from top to bottom including the core, which is rich in bioflavenoids. Cut each quarter into smaller pieces and put into blender. Rinse parsley and add to blender along with the lemon, peeled garlic, ginger, water, and honey if desired. You can also throw in kale or spinach if you like for extra anti-inflammatory nutrition.

Blend at high speed until consistency is smooth and enjoy!

4. CASHEW CHEESE

1 c cashews (soaked if possible)
1 clove garlic
1 tbs fresh lemon juice
½ tsp sea salt

Combine in a blender with just enough water to almost cover the cashews. Blend like crazy.

5. YUMMY AVOCADO SANDWICH

Ezekiel or other sprouted grain or flourless bread toasted
½ avocado, sliced
1 small tomato, sliced
1 c salad greens (kale, spinach, or your favorite mixture)
¼ small onion thinly sliced
¼ c apple cider or balsamic vinegar
1 tsp Bragg's liquid amino
splash of fresh lemon juice
1 pinch each of garlic granules, onion granules, ground cumin, and smoked paprika

Combine balsamic vinegar, Bragg's liquid amino, pepper, cumin, garlic granules, onion granules, smoked paprika, or spice mixture of your choice, to taste, in a small jar with lid and shake well to blend.

Toast bread. Slice avocado and place on one slice of bread to cover. Drizzle a teaspoon of the vinegar and spice mixture over the avocado slices. Place onion, tomato slices, and greens on top of avocado, and drizzle another teaspoon of the dressing. Top with second slice of bread and enjoy. You can use the remaining dressing to make a side salad with the extra greens.

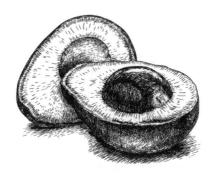

6. BAKED SWEET POTATO "FRIES"

◇◇

   1 large sweet potato, scrubbed
   1 tsp black pepper
   1 tsp garlic powder

Preheat oven to 425 degrees and line a baking sheet with parchment paper.

Peel or keep potato skin. Cut into wedges and toss in a bowl with pepper and garlic powder. Place them spaced apart in a single layer on the baking sheet.

Bake 25–30 minutes or until tender and browned on the edges. Serve immediately.

7. "BETTER-THAN-TUNA" SALAD

◇◇

   1 15-oz can of salt-free chickpeas, drained and rinsed
   ½ c cashew mayo*
   ⅓ c diced celery
   ¼ c diced red onion
   ¼ c diced red pepper
   ¼ c fresh or frozen corn
   1 tbs pumpkin seeds (soaked 1 hour)
   1 tbs fresh lemon juice
   1 tsp Bragg's liquid aminos
   1 tbs Dijon mustard
   2 tbs capers (drained)
   ⅓ c chopped celery
   ¼ c chopped green onion or red onion
   ¼ c chopped red bell pepper

½ tsp black pepper

¼ tsp cayenne pepper (or more to taste)

1 tbs fresh dill

Cashew Mayo

1 c raw unsalted cashews soaked for 30 minutes in hot water

½ c water

1 tbs Braggs liquid aminos

2 tbs lemon juice or apple cider vinegar

Makes 1 cup which will last in covered container in refrigerator for up to one week. Will use ½ cup.

Soak cashews and pumpkin seeds in hot water in two separate containers for 30 minutes before starting recipe, or overnight separately in warm water. Make the cashew mayo using the soaked cashews. Place chickpeas in a bowl and mash them with a fork. Add in ½ cup of the cashew mayo and stir into the chickpea mixture. Finally add in all the remaining ingredients and enjoy with lettuce cups or on toasted bread.

8. CORN RICE SALAD WITH AVOCADO

1 tsp garlic powder

3 c leftover cooked brown rice or quinoa

2 c roasted corn kernels (thawed if frozen)

1 bunch scallions, thinly sliced (greens only)

½ c chopped cilantro

½ tsp black pepper or red pepper flakes

½ c nutritional yeast

1 large avocado, diced

2 tbs freshly squeezed lemon juice

2 tbs balsamic vinegar

Combine all ingredients except lemon juice, Braggs liquid aminos, balsamic vinegar, and avocados. Add the avocados, juice, Braggs liquid aminos, balsamic vinegar and fold in. Cover and refrigerate until ready to serve.

9. RAW VEGAN PESTO

8 oz fresh organic basil

¾ c raw pumpkin seeds, sunflower seeds or walnuts

½ c Bragg's nutritional yeast flakes

1 tsp sea salt or to taste

4 tbs fresh squeezed lemon juice

5–8 cloves garlic

⅓ c veggie broth

Add seeds, nutritional yeast, garlic cloves, salt, veggie broth, and lemon juice. Rinse, pick, and pack basil leaves into the food processor. Pulse and process for 3–4 minutes, making sure all ingredients are well mixed. Makes about 1 to 1½ cup pesto to use as dip, spread, or with pasta.

10. SIMPLE TOMATO SAUCE

¼ c sun dried tomatoes

1 small red tomato

1 small clove garlic

1–2 basil leaves

½ tsp sea salt

Cut the tomato into four pieces and squeeze out the seeds and the liquid. Put in blender and blend away until smooth consistency.

11. LENTIL SOUP

2 c lentils

4 c water or vegetable broth

2 tbs finely grated ginger (optional)

3 large garlic cloves

1 tbs cumin

1 tbs smoked paprika

1 tsp coriander

1 tsp apple cider vinegar

1 tbs fresh lemon juice

3 tbs Braggs amino or to taste

½ c chopped carrots

½ c chopped celery

1 c chopped onion

½ c fresh parsley

Put lentils and water in large pot with ginger, garlic, onions, and celery and bring to a boil. Add other ingredients including half of the parsley, lower heat and simmer for 25 minutes. Remove from heat and sprinkle remaining parsley as a garnish.

12. SOUPE KANDIA

2 c chopped onion

1 c chopped green bell pepper

1 c sliced celery

1 c diced tomatoes

2 c sliced okra (fresh or frozen)

¼ c gumbo file powder

¼ c garbanzo bean flour (adds protein and flavor)

4 c vegetable broth (more or less based on desired thickness)

1 tsp salt
2 tbs garlic powder
1 tsp cumin
1 tsp paprika
Cayenne pepper to taste

Using ¼ cup of the vegetable broth, sauté chopped onion, green pepper, and celery in Dutch kettle or large pot using medium heat until it softens and starts to brown.

Add spices, 3 cups vegetable broth, stir and cover.

In a small, non-stick skillet, sauté garbanzo bean flour, and when brown add gumbo file, ¼ cup of vegetable broth, and stir while bubbling to make the roux.

Add roux and tomatoes to large pot.

Using same small skillet and another ¼ cup of vegetable broth, add okra and brown. When slightly browned and not "slimy," add to pot. Reduce heat cover and simmer for 30 minutes until flavors blend. Taste and adjust spices as desired and serve over brown rice.

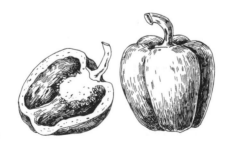

13. THIEBOUDIENNE

1 c chopped onion

1 c chopped parsley (save 1 tbs for garnish)

4 cloves garlic chopped

5 c water

1 small–medium yucca root peeled and cut in 4-5 pieces

2 medium–large carrots cut in half

1 medium sweet potato or small summer squash cut in quarters

1 diced jalapeño or habanero (remove seeds)

1 small eggplant cut in quarters

1 c zucchini

½ small cabbage

1 c cauliflower florets

½ c tomato paste

1 c diced tomatoes

1 can garbanzo beans

3 dried tamarind pods (adds tangy flavor!)

Lime wedges

Spices

2 tsp black pepper

1 tsp red pepper flakes

1 tsp turmeric

1 tsp ground cloves

2 bay leaves

2 tbs garlic powder

2 tsp salt or Braggs liquid amino to taste

Sauté onion, parsley, and garlic in ¼ cup water until lightly browned. Add rest of water along with tomato paste, diced tomatoes, and spices and bring to a boil. Add yucca, sweet potato or summer squash, and carrot and boil for 5 minutes. Reduce heat, add tamarind pods, garbanzo beans, jalapeño pepper, cabbage, and eggplant and simmer on medium to low heat for 25–30 minutes to allow flavors to blend. When the yucca is easily pierced with a fork, add the cabbage, cauliflower, and zucchini and simmer for another 10 minutes. Serve over brown rice and garnish with the reserved fresh parsley and a lime wedge.

Bouillon cubes that contain MSG and powdered chicken are traditionally used. Substitution here includes turmeric, salt, black pepper, garlic powder, onion powder, ground cloves and bay leaf.

14. OIL-FREE INDIAN VEGETABLE CURRY

1 c cubed potatoes
½ c sliced carrots
½ c green peas
½ c button mushrooms
1 c cauliflower florets
1 c cut green beans
1 c shredded cabbage
½ tsp mustard seeds or powder
1 tsp Cumin seeds
½ c onion finely chopped
2 or 3 large garlic cloves pureed
1 tsp turmeric powder
1 tsp curry powder
1 tsp red pepper flakes (or more to taste)
⅔ c plain soy or cashew yogurt
1 tsp cornstarch
2 tsp coconut sugar or other sugar
2 tbs liquid aminos or to taste
3 tbs fresh cilantro (coriander) or bay leaves to top (optional)
Water

Prep first seven vegetables. Place the potatoes and carrots in a pot of boiling water, with enough water to cover all the vegetables. After about 3 minutes, add the remaining five vegetables and boil until nearly tender but still firm. Drain well and set aside.

Put the soy yogurt and cornstarch in a small bowl, whisk to mix well and set aside.

In a large skillet or pan, heat ¼ cup water to a boil and add the cumin seeds and mustard seeds or powder; reduce heat to medium and stir frequently until the seeds begin to soften and the mixture begins to darken. Add the onion and garlic and continue to "stir fry" for another 2 to 3 minutes adding a little extra water when it starts to dry. Then add the turmeric, curry, red pepper flakes, stir for another 2 to 3 minutes, adding a little water if needed to prevent burning until spice mixture is a golden brown.

Add in the drained vegetables and lower heat. Stir to coat vegetables with the spice mixture, add the sugar and salt (or liquid aminos) and gradually stir in the yogurt/cornstarch mixture. Sprinkle the fresh cilantro or place fresh bay leaves on top, reduce heat and simmer to allow flavors to blend. I love it with brown rice or quinoa!

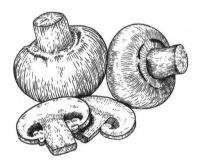

15. SPICY BLACK BEANS

4 c dried black beans (soaked overnight)

2½ quarts (10 c) water

1 tablespoon dried oregano

3 bay leaves

3 large sage leaves

2 teaspoons sea salt or Braggs liquid aminos

2 yellow onions, chopped

2 jalapeños, seeds discarded

6 cloves crushed garlic

2 tablespoons chili powder

1–2 teaspoons chipotle powder

1 tbs cumin powder

Juice of 1 lime

Chopped fresh cilantro for garnish

Add rehydrated beans, oregano, bay leaves, and sage to pot with 10 cups of water. Bring beans to a boil and reduce heat to a simmer for 45 minutes.

Remove bay leaves and sage from the pot; add in onions, peppers, and spices. Salt to taste or add liquid amino for a lower sodium option. Cook for another hour or so until beans are cooked through and reach desired tenderness. Add lime and cilantro and serve.

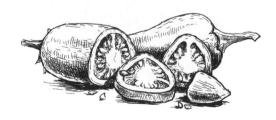

16. CHIPOTLE VEGAN ENCHILADAS

Chipotle Sauce:

2 cloves chopped garlic

1 tsp cumin

½ tsp chili powder

¼ tsp smoked paprika

¼ tsp black pepper

¼ c chipotle chilis in adobo sauce

1¼ c veggie broth

1 c crushed canned tomatoes

1 tbs liquid aminos

Filling:

½ c diced sweet potato

½ c fresh or frozen corn

1 can beans drained

1½ c shredded vegan cheddar or mozzarella cheese

1 tbs onion powder

1 tbs garlic powder

1 tsp liquid aminos

10-12 corn tortillas

Preheat oven to 400F. Place diced potatoes on baking sheet and and bake for 30 minutes. Combine baked potatoes with ½ c vegan cheese, corn and beans in a separate bowl with onion powder, garlic powder and liquid aminos. Reduce oven temperature to 350F.

Chipotle Sauce:

While potatoes are baking, make your chipotle sauce. First heat your pot, add ¼ cup of veggie broth, and once it is hot, sauté garlic for 30 seconds. Add the cumin, black pepper, chili powder, and smoked paprika. Stir to combine, and cook for 30 seconds. Add the chipotle chilis, the remaining broth, crushed tomatoes, liquid aminos, and stir to combine. Bring chipotle sauce to a boil and then reduce to a simmer until sauce is thickened or about 5 minutes. Put sauce in blender on medium speed until smooth and set aside.

Pour enough chipotle sauce to cover the bottom of an 8"x11" baking dish. Assemble your enchiladas by making a line the center of each tortilla with your filling mixture. Tuck one side under the mixture and roll to hold the mixture inside and place seam down in the dish.

Once all enchiladas are placed in the dish pour the rest of your sauce on top and any leftover filling on the sides. Sprinkle with remaining shredded cheese and bake for 20 minutes. Serve hot.

17. PICO DE GALLO

2 c diced fresh tomatoes
½ c fresh cilantro
1 small onion chopped
1 medium size jalapeno pepper, seeds removed and diced
1 tbs lime or lemon juice
1 tsp sea salt
1 tsp garlic powder
½ tsp ground cumin

Mix all ingredients in a medium sized bowl, adjust spice to taste, and refrigerate 2–3 hours before serving. It will be even better the next day. Sprinkle over tacos, enchiladas, beans, vegetables, or use in recipes for an extra flavor kick!

18. SPICY BLACK-EYED PEAS

1½ c dried black-eyed peas (rinsed and soaked overnight)

1 small onion sliced

3 cloves of garlic diced or pressed

½ c celery sliced

½ c carrots thickly sliced

½ c diced tomatoes

4 c low-sodium veggie broth; set aside 3 tbs for sauté

1 tbs cumin powder

2 tbs smoked paprika

1 tbs apple cider vinegar

3 tbs Braggs liquid aminos or to taste

3 tbs vegetable broth

Sauté onion and garlic in 3 tbs vegetable broth until translucent or slightly browned. Add remaining broth and bring to a boil.

Add peas and bring back to boil. Add cumin, smoked paprika, liquid aminos, diced tomatoes, and vinegar. Stir and reduce heat, cover, and cook on medium heat until peas soften and liquid starts to thicken. Add carrots and celery and cook until tender.

19. SAUTÉED COLLARD GREENS

1 c vegetable broth or water

1 small onion, halved and sliced and cut in strips

1 bunch collard greens, stems removed, washed (or kale)

1 c sliced cherry tomatoes

1 tbs lemon juice

1 tbs apple cider vinegar

1 tsp black pepper

1 tbs garlic powder (or chopped fresh garlic)

1 tsp sea salt or Braggs liquid aminos to taste

In a large skillet, heat a half cup of broth or water, add onions, half of the tomatoes, and sauté for about 5 minutes. Add rest of the broth or water, lemon juice, vinegar, pepper, garlic powder, and salt or liquid aminos and and stir to blend. Then add the greens, remainder of tomatoes, and stir for 2–3 minutes to make sure they all are coated with the liquid and spices. Cover and simmer on low heat for another 15 minutes.

20. CLARA'S VEGAN CORNBREAD

1 c yellow cornmeal

1½ c oat (gluten free) or wheat flour

1 tbs baking powder

1 tsp sea salt

⅓ c unsweetened apple sauce

1½ tbs maple syrup

3 tbs almond butter

1 c unsweetened almond or other plant milk

Lightly oil an 8x8 inch pan and preheat your oven to 400 degrees.

Combine dry ingredients in a large bowl and stir to mix well. Add maple syrup, apple sauce, and almond butter to bowl and stir to mix. Finally add the almond milk to the batter and stir well. Pour batter into pan and bake for 30 minutes or until it browns. You can check by inserting a toothpick which should come out clean when it's done.

Cut into small squares and store in refrigerator in a sealed bag or container to keep moist. That is if you don't eat the whole pan!

21. VEGAN BROCCOLI QUINOA

3 c cooked quinoa

5 c raw broccoli, cut into small florets and stems

3 medium garlic cloves

⅔ c sliced or slivered almonds, toasted

⅓ c vegan parmesan or nutritional yeast

¼ c veggie broth

¼ c coconut milk or cashew cream

Slivered basil

Sliced avocado

1 tsp dried red pepper flakes

Heat the quinoa and set aside.

Now barely cook the broccoli by pouring ¾ c water into a large pot and bringing it to a simmer. Add a big pinch of salt and stir in the broccoli. Cover and cook for a minute, just long enough to take the raw edge off. Transfer the broccoli to a strainer and run under cold water until it stops cooking. Set aside.

To make the broccoli pesto, puree two cups of the cooked broccoli, the garlic, ½ cup of the almonds, vegan parmesan (or brewer's yeast), salt, and lemon juice in a food processor. Drizzle in the olive oil and cream and pulse until smooth.

Just before serving, toss the quinoa and remaining broccoli florets with about ½ of the broccoli pesto. Taste and adjust if needed; you might want to add more of the pesto a bit at a time, or you might want a bit more salt or an added squeeze of lemon juice. Turn out onto a serving platter and top with the remaining almonds. Garnish with sliced avocado slices sprinkled with red pepper flakes and the slivered basil.

22. BAKED CORNMEAL ONION RINGS

1 large or 2 medium sweet onion

4 c almond or other plant milk

2 tbs plus 2 tsp apple cider vinegar

¾ c raw sesame seeds

½ c cornmeal

½ c ground raw pepitas

1 tsp smoked paprika

1 tsp garlic powder

½ tsp dried oregano

¼ tsp turmeric powder

½ tsp sea salt

1 tsp black pepper

Mix vinegar with almond milk to create a vegan buttermilk. Set aside. Slice onions into half-inch-thick circles and soak for 4 hours.

Heat oven to 450. In a medium size bowl, combine 1 cup of the vegan buttermilk with the sesame seeds, mix into a batter, then set aside.

In another shallow bowl, combine cornmeal, ground pepitas, and spices in a bowl or shallow dish and also set aside.

One by one, separate onion rings, dip in batter and coat well. Then coat with cornmeal-pepita-spice mixture. Place on a parchment lined cookie sheet. Flip after baking for 10 minutes and bake for another 15-20 minutes. Enjoy while fresh and crispy.

23. RAW CASHEW CHOCOLATE CHEESECAKE

2½ c raw cashews

1 tsp pure vanilla extract

⅓ c raw cacao powder

½ c pure maple syrup or honey

¼ c + 1 tbs almond butter

¼ c lemon juice

½ c water

Pinch of salt

Put cashews in a bowl and cover with water. Soak overnight or at least 6–8 hours. Drain, spread on paper towel, and pat completely dry.

Crust:

1 c pitted dates

2 c raw almonds

Pinch of salt

¼ tsp pure vanilla extract

1 or 2 tsp water, if needed

Line a round 9-inch springform pan with parchment paper and set aside; this makes it easy to remove from pan. Combine all crust ingredients except water in a food processor (do not blend) until fine crumbles form. If the mixture is too dry, add the water. Press the crust mixture into the parchment paper covered bottom of the pan. Cover and freeze until ready to use.

Filling:

Combine all ingredients (including the ¼ cup water) in a high-speed food processor or Vitamix and process for 5 minutes. Stop to scrape down the sides, and process for 1–2 more minutes. Repeat the scraping step if necessary to get all the mixture blended. Pour into your prepared crust or use a graham cracker crust.

Put the cheesecake in the freezer for 15–20 minutes to set, then enjoy! You can store it in the freezer for up to 2 weeks. Just thaw for 20 minutes before serving.

Tip: Blend a handful of strawberries with a tablespoon of maple syrup or other sweetener to make delicious and colorful drizzle to add before serving.

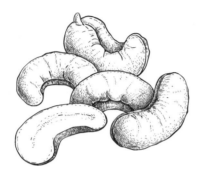

24. ZOELA'S APPLE CRISP

Fruit
4 c peeled sliced apples (Honeycrisp, Pink Lady work well) or
    any fresh fruit or berries
2 tbs maple syrup
1 tbs tapioca starch or gluten-free flour
2 tbs lemon juice
½ tsp ground cinnamon

Crisp
½ c almond or oat flour
⅓ c rolled oats
½ c roughly chopped walnuts or pecans
2 tbs creamy unsalted almond butter
4 tbs maple syrup
pinch of sea salt (optional)

Preheat oven to 350 degrees. Put sliced apples into an 8" x 8" baking pan. Sprinkle tapioca starch and cinnamon over apples, add maple syrup and lemon juice and toss to mix well.

Topping
Put almond or oat flour, oats, chopped walnuts, and sea salt in a large bowl and stir to mix. Add almond butter, maple syrup, and salt and mix well. Sprinkle topping over fruit to cover evenly.

Bake for 40 minutes or until topping is nice and brown. Let cool and serve. Great with vegan ice cream!

25. ABE'S HEART-Y BREAD

This final recipe is a bonus. I could not find a commercial gluten-free whole grain bread that had low salt and high taste. I hesitated to include it because baking bread is not simple or quick, but this bread is so delicious and full of healthy whole ingredients, great texture, and taste that I want to share. It's a little reminder that the best things often take time.

Soak:
3 tbs pumpkin or sunflower seeds

3 tbs red quinoa

3 tbs oats

Soak these ingredients in ⅓ c water for 6 hours.

Wet:
2 c warm water or plant milk

2¼ tsp instant yeast

3 tbs maple syrup

¼ c ground flax seeds

¼ c chia seeds

Add maple syrup in warm water and then add in yeast. Let sit for 10 minutes while yeast activates.

After yeast is activated, add flax meal, chia seeds, and soaked seeds/oats to yeast mixture. Let sit for 5–10 minutes.

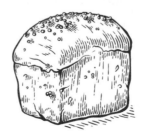

Dry:
½ c cornmeal
½ c millet flour
½ c brown rice flour
2¼ c oat flour
3 tbs tapioca starch
1 tbs psyllium husk powder
1 tbs salt

Mix dry ingredients together and add in the wet mixture.

Using a stand mixer or your hands knead the mixture together for 4-5 minutes until well combined.

Line a loaf pan with parchment paper and spread the dough mixture inside with a spatula. Once mixture is spread evenly cover with a damp towel in a warm area and let the dough rise for 1-2 hours until doubled in size.

When the dough has doubled in size remove the towel and place the loaf into the preheated oven at 410F for 45-55 minutes until the top is golden.

Once loaf is done, take the pan out and rest for 10 minutes before removing bread from the loaf pan.

After removing the bread let it cool entirely before slicing. (Approximately 2-3 hours)

Slice the bread and store in an airtight container for up to 4 days or freeze in a bag. Enjoy!

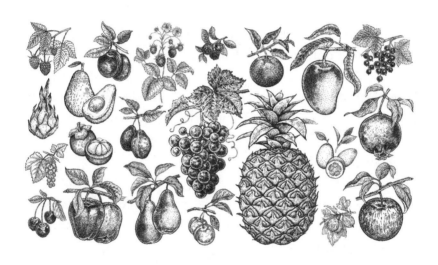

Acknowledgments

I WANT TO THANK ALL OF THE KIND and generous souls who encouraged this work. I am humbled by your confidence in me and grateful for every act and expression of support.

To my family: daughters Tembi Locke and Attica Locke—I couldn't have asked for better mentors on this journey. Your example of hard work, curiosity, fearlessness, and open hearts which drove your own excellence as writers and creative spirits has been more inspiring than you will ever know. Thanks to my grandchildren, Zoela and Clara, and my children of the heart, Michela Aguirre, Yvonne Aguirre, and Arthur Flanagan, for their patience in the face of too much unsolicited dietary advice. I thank my husband, Abe Seck, for his consistent support and for giving me the "you can do this" when I needed it most. Love and thanks to my extended family: "sister/cousins" Pamiel Gaskin, whose story I shared, Cheryl Stephens and Dr. Lennette Benjamin; cousins Dr. Kevin Smith who graciously consented to a video of his personal food journey, and his brother, humanitarian/activist Dr. Cedrick Smith whose passion and generous spirit are rare indeed. I have been uplifted by our whole family village.

To the enormously talented literary and publishing veterans who have guided me by investing their time, counsel, and industry expertise: Marah Stets, Cherise Fisher, and Fauzia Burke, who all opened doors to the resources I needed through their introductions, and Melody R. Guy, developmental editor extraordinaire; I will always remember your enthusiasm for this work and generosity in supporting it. Many of the recipes in this book were the product of my collaboration with chef Karen Fernandez, aka "Vegana Tejana," who made the process more fun than I could ever imagine, and more delicious as well! My special appreciation goes to Brooke Warner and the She Writes Press team for providing opportunities for new voices like my own among women writers.

To the wonderful community of physicians who are adding nutrition-based therapies and patient education to their practices, holistic health care providers, farmers, food justice advocates, environmental and animal rights activists, and the entire plant-based food community: I am honored to join ranks and lend support to all of you. With great love and commitment, you are doing incredibly important work.

Endnotes

Introduction

1. Robert Preidt, CBS News Healthday, January 27, 2017. Based on American Heart Association report, "Heart Disease and Stroke Statistics—2017"

2. Black Women's Health Imperative Staff, "Heart Disease in Black Women: The Big Issue You May Not Know About," Black Women's Health Imperative, February 12, 2018, https://bwhi.org/2018/02/12/heart-disease-black-women-big-issue-might-not-know/.

3. US Department of Health and Human Services, Office of Minority Health, February 14, 2020, https://minorityhealth.hhs.gov/omh/browse.aspx?lvl=4&lvlid=19.

4. Centers for Disease Control and Prevention. *National Diabetes Statistics Report, 2020*, Atlanta, GA: Centers for Disease Control and Prevention, US Department of Health and Human Services; 2020.

5. Office of Minority Health, US Department of Health and Human Services, "Diabetes and African Americans, Source: National Healthcare Quality and Disparities Reports," December 05, 2019, https://minorityhealth.hhs.gov/omh/browse.aspx?lvl=4&lvlid=18.

6. Lin, J., Thompson et al. "Projection of the future diabetes burden in the United States through 2060." *Population Health Metrics* 16, no. 9 (2018): https://doi.org/10.1186/s12963-018-0166-4.

PART I
Chapter 2
7. Lisa Elaine Held, "The Ultimate Summary of the China Study: Here's What You Need to Know," Well + Good, published September 23, 2011; updated August 9, 2018,https://www.wellandgood.com/china-study-cheat-sheet-10-things-you-need-to-know/.

8. Caldwell B. Esselstyn,Jr., M.D., *Prevent and Reverse Heart Disease: The Revolutionary, Scientifically Proven, Nutrition-Based Cure* (Penguin Books, 2007), 87–88.

9. Loma Linda University, "Adventist Health Study Overview," September 2011, https://publichealth.llu.edu/sites/publichealth.llu.edu/files/docs/sph-ahs-overview.pdf.

10. PubMed Central (PMC), Archive of the US National Institutes of Health's National Library of Medicine (NIH/NLM), "Meat consumption and mortality—results from the European Prospective Investigation into Cancer (EPIC) and Nutrition," published March 7, 2013, https://www.ncbi.nlm.nih.gov/pmc/articles/PMC3599112/.

11. Alice G. Walton, Senior Contributor, Forbes Magazine, "Swap Your Diet, Swap Your Cancer Risk, New Study Finds," Apr 28, 2015, https://www.forbes.com/sites/alicegwalton/2015/04/28/swap-your-diet-swap-your-cancer-risk-new-study-finds/#7350ffd128db.

Chapter 3

12. Caldwell B. Esselstyn, Jr., M.D., *Prevent and Reverse Heart Disease: The Revolutionary, Scientifically Proven, Nutrition-Based Cure*, (Penguin Books: 2007), 67–75.

13. Caldwell B. Esselstyn, Jr., M.D., *Prevent and Reverse Heart Disease: The Revolutionary, Scientifically Proven, Nutrition-Based Cure*, (Penguin Books: 2007), 75.

14. Dean Ornish, M.D., *Dr. Dean Ornish's Program for Reversing Heart Disease*, (Random House: 1990), 261.

15. Dean Ornish, M.D., *Dr. Dean Ornish's Program for Reversing Heart Disease*, (Random House: 1990), 139–251.

Chapter 4

16. Michael Moss, Author and Pulitzer Prize Winner, "The Extraordinary Science of Junk Food," *New York Times Magazine*, February 2, 2013, http://www.nytimes.com/2013/02/24/magazine/the-extraordinary-science-of-junk-food.html?pagewanted=all&_r=2.

17. Daniel Lieberman, "Evolution's Sweet Tooth" *New York Times*, June 5, 2012; author of *The Evolution of the Human Head*, http://www.nytimes.com/2012/06/06/opinion/evolutions-sweet-tooth.html.

18. Dr. Mark Hyman, "Three Hidden Ways Wheat Makes You Fat," February 2, 2013, https://drhyman.com/blog/2012/02/13/three-hidden-ways-wheat-makes-you-fat/.

19. Food Addiction Research Education, http://foodaddiction research.org/resources.

Chapter 5

20. Environmental Working Group; nonprofit, nonpartisan organization dedicated to protecting human health and the environment. "Dirty Dozen" and "Clean Fifteen" annual produce list: http://www.ewg.org/about-us#.WWqTw9Pys0R.

PART II
Chapter 6

21. Rachel Metzer Warren MS, "Seasonal Eating for Your Body," Cleveland Clinic Wellness, June 15, 2010, http://www.cleveland clinicwellness.com/food/SeasonalEating/Pages/Seasonal Eating forYourBody.aspx.

Chapter 7

22. Lisa Beres, "Guide to Healthy Sweeteners", February 28, 2020, https://earth911.com/how-and-buy/guide-healthy-sweeteners/.

23. Jay Hoffman and Michael Falvo, "Protein – Which is Best?", International Society of Sports Nutrition Symposium, June 2004, Las Vegas NV USA, Journal of Sports Science and Medicine, September 2004, https://www.ncbi.nlm.nih.gov/pmc/articles/PMC3905294/.

24. Alisa Rutherford-Fortunati, "10 Protein-Packed Plants", October 31, 2011, www.gentleworld.org.

Chapter 8

25. John Staughton (BASc, BFA), "12 Surprising Benefits of Chipotle," Organic Facts, updated February 05, 2020, https://www.organicfacts. net/chipotle.html.

26. E. Richard Brown, *Medicine Men: Medicine and Capitalism in America*, (University of California Press: 1979).

Resources

BOOKS

Afro-Vegan: Farm-Fresh African, Caribbean, and Southern Flavors Remixed, Bryant Terry, 9781607745310, Ten Speed Press, 2014

Ageless Vegan: The Secret to Living a Long and Healthy Plant-Based Life, Tracye McQuirter, 9780738220208, Da Capo Lifelong Books, June 12, 2018

Carbon Yoga: The Vegan Metamorphosis, Dr. Sailesh Rao, 9781533019295, A Climate Healers Publication, 2016.

Pig Tales, Barry Estabrook, 9780393240245, W.W. Norton & Company, May 4, 2015

Plant-Based on a Budget: Delicious Vegan Recipes for Under $30 a Week, in Less Than 30 Minutes a Meal, Toni Okamoto and Dr. Michael Greger, BenBella Books Inc, May 14, 2019

The Alzheimer's Solution: A Breakthrough Program to Prevent and Reverse the Symptoms of Cognitive Decline at Every Age,

Dr. Ayesha Sherzai and Dr. Dean Sherzai, 9780062666482, Harper Collins Publishers, January 29, 2019

"The Blue Zones of Happiness: Lessons From the World's Happiest People" Dan Buettner, 9781426218484, National Geographic Partners, October 3, 2017

The End of Heart Disease: The Eat to Live Plan to Prevent and Reverse Heart Disease, Joel Fuhrman, 9780062249364, HarperOne, March 27, 2018

The Engine 2 Cookbook, Rip Esselstyn and Jane Esselstyn, 9781455591206, Hatchette Book Group, December 2017

The How Not to Die Cookbook, Michael Greger, M.D., FACLM, 9781250127761, Flatiron Books, December 2017

The Plant-Based Solution: America's Healthy Heart Doc's Plan to Power Your Health, Joel K. Kahn, 9781683644651, Sounds True, February 1, 2020

What the Health, Kip Andersen and Eunice Wong, 9781946885524, BenBella Books, Inc, February 22, 2017

FILMS

Concealed Cruelty, film by Mercy for Animals
http://pigabuse.mercyforanimals.org/

Forks Over Knives, synopsis and download; also on Netflix
https://www.forksoverknives.com/synopsis/#gs.z5jWFmI

Vegucated, film about the realities of eating animal products, available on Netflix, iTunes, or Amazon
http://www.getvegucated.com/the-film/what-people-are-saying/lives-changed/

Food, Inc., documentary by Robert Kenner, April 2008 on the takeover of the American food chain by huge corporations, issues of animal cruelty, health, and food safety

ARTICLES, STUDIES AND BLOG POSTS

James McWilliams, "PSTD in the Slaughterhouse," *Texas Observer*, February 2012
https://www.texasobserver.org/ptsd-in-the-slaughterhouse/

"7 Ways to Eat Good on a Hood Budget" by Stic of Dead Prez in blog post by Toni Okamoto,
https://plantbasedonabudget.com/7-ways-to-eat-good-while-on-a-hood-budget-by-stic-of-dead-prez/

"Pharmaceutical Industry gets High on Fat Profits," Richard Anderson, Business reporter, BBC News, November 6, 2014
http://www.bbc.com/news/business-28212223

"Livestock's Long Shadow: Environmental Issues and Options" is a United Nations report, released by the Food and Agriculture Organization of the United Nations (FAO) on 29 November 2006

Adventist Health Studies https://nutritionfacts.org/topics/adventist-health-studies/

"Protein—Which is Best?," Jay Hoffman and Michael Falvo, *Journal of Health and Sports Science Medicine*, September 1, 2004, study presented at the International Society of Sports Nutrition Symposium, Las Vegas NV, June 2005

Loma Linda University, "Adventist Health Study Overview," September 2011 https://publichealth.llu.edu/sites/publichealth.llu.edu/files/docs/sph-ahs-overview.pdf

"Veggie-based diets could save 8 million lives by 2050 and cut global warming," Oxford University news article, https://www.ox.ac.uk/news/2016-03-22-veggie-based-diets-could-save-8-million-lives-2050-and-cut-global-warming, March 22, 2016

Source research paper:

"Analysis and Valuation of Health and Climate Change Cobenefits of Dietary Change," Dr. Marco Springmann, lead researcher, Oxford University study, published in the Proceedings of National Academy of Sciences Journal, March 21, 2016, https://www.pnas.org/content/113/15/4146

About the Author

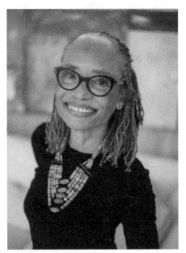

photo © Grady Carter

SHERRA AGUIRRE founded and led a successful business for thirty-five years, winning national awards for entrepreneurship, innovation, and service excellence. She sold the business in 2016 to focus on her passion for healthy diet and lifestyle.

Now in her seventies, Aguirre describes herself as high energy, in better overall health, and in many ways more fit than in her thirties or forties. She has practiced meditation and yoga daily for more than twenty-five years, and for many years has researched and read extensively about diet and lifestyle as the most important factors for achieving and maintaining good health. By adopting a whole plant-based diet, she improved overall heart health and eliminated symptoms of hypertension despite a significant family history of heart attack, stroke, and high blood pressure. She is passionate about empowering others to maintain vibrancy and good health throughout their lifetimes.

As a health enthusiast, environmentalist, and food justice advocate, Aguirre writes about the healing qualities of compassion, simplicity, and gratitude, and the ripple effect vegan eating can have on individuals, families, and communities. Sherra is married with two daughters—Tembi Locke, actor, speaker, screenwriter, and New *New York Times* best-selling author; and Attica Locke, multiple award-winning novelist, *New York Times* best-selling author and screen writer/producer. Visit Sherra online:

www.sherraaguirre.com

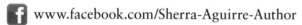 www.facebook.com/Sherra-Aguirre-Author

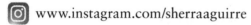 www.instagram.com/sherraaguirre

www.linkedin.com/in/sherra-aguirre

Selected Titles From She Writes Press

She Writes Press is an independent publishing
company founded to serve women writers everywhere.
Visit us at www.shewritespress.com.

Raw by Bella Mahaya Carter. $16.95, 978-1-63152-345-8. In an effort to holistically cure her chronic stomach problems, Bella Mahaya Carter adopted a 100 percent raw, vegan diet—a first step on a quest that ultimately dragged her, kicking and screaming, into spiritual adulthood.

The Great Healthy Yard Project: Our Yards, Our Children, Our Responsibility by Diane Lewis, MD. $24.95, 978-1-938314-86-5. A comprehensive look at the ways in which we are polluting our drinking water and how it's putting our children's future at risk—and what we can do to turn things around.

Renewable: One Woman's Search for Simplicity, Faithfulness, and Hope by Eileen Flanagan. $16.95, 978-1-63152-968-9. At age forty-nine, Eileen Flanagan had an aching feeling that she wasn't living up to her youthful ideals or potential, so she started trying to change the world—and in doing so, she found the courage to change her life.

Think Better. Live Better. 5 Steps to Create the Life You Deserve by Francine Huss. $16.95, 978-1-938314-66-7. With the help of this guide, readers will learn to cultivate more creative thoughts, realign their mindset, and gain a new perspective on life.

Hedgebrook Cookbook: Celebrating Radical Hospitality by Denise Barr & Julie Rosten. $24.95, 978-1-93831-422-3. Delectable recipes and inspiring writing, straight from Hedgebrook's farmhouse table to yours.